DETOX
FOR LIFE

D0531153

CAROL VORDERMAN'S
DETOX FOR LIFE
THE 28-DAY DETOX DIET AND BEYOND

Carol Vorderman
With Ko Chohan
Written by Anita Bean

Virgin BOOKS

Published by Virgin Books 2009

4 6 8 10 9 7 5 3

First published in Great Britain in 2001 by
Virgin Books
Random House, 20 Vauxhall Bridge Road,
London SW1V 2SA

www.virginbooks.com
www.randomhouse.co.uk

Addresses for companies within The Random House Group Limited can be found at: www.
randomhouse.co.uk/offices.htm

The Random House Group Limited Reg. No. 954009

A CIP catalogue record for this book
is available from the British Library

ISBN 9780753516812

The Random House Group Limited supports The Forest Stewardship Council (FSC), the
leading international forest certification organisation. All our titles that are printed on
Greenpeace approved FSC certified paper carry the FSC logo. Our paper procurement
policy can be found at: www.randomhouse.co.uk/environment

Mixed Sources
Product group from well-managed
forests and other controlled sources
www.fsc.org Cert no. TT-COC-002139
© 1996 Forest Stewardship Council

Typeset by Palimpsest Book Production Limited, Grangemouth, Stirlingshire
Printed in the UK by CPI Bookmarque, Croydon, CR0 4TD

CONTENTS

Checking with your Doctor

Before starting this or any detox diet programme, you should consult your doctor. In particular this should be done with regard to any allergies you have to any of the foods, drinks, products, supplements or any other recommendations contained in this programme. This detox diet may not be suitable for everyone. Pregnant women should be especially careful and ensure that their doctor advises that the detox diet is suitable for them. If you are taking any medication or have any medical condition, you should check with your doctor first.

While the authors have made every effort to ensure that the information contained within this book is as accurate and up to date as possible, it is advisory only and should not be used as an alternative to seeking specialist medical advice. The authors and publisher cannot be held responsible for actions that may be taken by a reader as a result of reliance on the information contained in this book, which are taken entirely at the reader's own risk.

INTRODUCTION

I came across the detox diet ten years ago. Since then, I've followed the 28 day diet roughly twice a year, usually straight after Christmas and just before the summer hols. It worked for me and for thousands and thousands of other people. I feel healthier, younger and free of those mornings when you wake up and the scales don't say what you want them to.

The facts are:
I'm over forty
I weigh myself only once every three months
I don't ever count calories
I don't go to a gym

BUT
I'm the same size I was when I was twenty – a size 8 to 10
I have more energy than I've ever had in my life
And I eat loads of food every day

All of this is thanks to the 28 day detox plan, which rewrites the rules that you and I have slavishly, and I believe wrongly, followed in so-called 'dieting' plans for years.

The detox is not about counting calories or fat units, it's about being aware of the kinds of food we are putting into our bodies. It's not about eating less it's about eating more.

So is it for you? Well, whatever age or sex you are, the detox is ideal if you want to:

- Lose weight
- Lose inches and bloat
- Change your shape

- Get rid of a lot of cellulite
- Stop feeling unhealthy, constantly tired or sluggish

Does it sound like it could help you? Well it's time to be honest, not with me, but with yourself. Answer these questions truthfully and make a list of all the things you've tried over the years.

How many 'diets' have you started? How many promised that you would 'Lose 10 pounds in a week' but didn't work?

How many books have you read about dieting? How many magazines do you buy that promise a magical slimming regime?

Do you get on the scales every day and end up disappointed? When was the last time you weighed yourself and were happy with the result?

Have you paid for an exercise bike or a six-month membership of a gym only to stop using it after the first week? How much did it cost? Why didn't you just walk past the front door and chuck some cash in instead?

Do you get fed up every day because you feel overweight and you can't get into clothes that you love?

How many times do you think about food in a day? How often do you feel guilty when you eat?

Are you honest? The answers are depressing aren't they? I know because I've done all of those things myself. I did them because I used to think that weight control was all about counting calories and denying myself things that I wanted to eat. I'm 5' 6" and a bit, and from my mid-twenties onwards I was always a dress size bigger than I wanted to be, but I wasn't able to shift the inches. I knew the calorific value of every product on a supermarket shelf. It didn't stop me from eating bad stuff but I knew it never the less. I weighed myself every day and I knew all the tricks. Do it first thing in the morning with no clothes on and put the scales inside the bath so that they say you weigh less (hard surfaces you see). If they said I'd put on a few pounds, I'd start the day feeling bad, swearing that I'd eat less.

All day I'd add up my calories in my head: toast, jam and cappuccino to start with. Baked potato and 'just a bit of chocolate', then by teatime I'd be way over my self-imposed allowance, be really fed up and decide not to have any tea (or dinner). But then of course I would have tea, and I'd go to bed really, really fed up with myself, get up the next morning and the whole thing would start all over again. Just getting on the scales would be enough to give a grey shadow to a day. Ridiculous really, but I guess it's been true for most of us at some time.

Then every now and again I'd get to the point where I thought 'No, I am going to do something now.' I'd read about some fad diet where you just eat cabbage for a week, try it for two days, something would go wrong and I'd end up fed up again. In fact I'd be even more fed up than I was before and off I'd go on the famous yo-yo.

But it was when I had my first baby that things started to get out of control. I couldn't lose the weight after I had Katie. I was 31 years old and I went up to a size 14. I felt old and sluggish and always dressed with jackets to hide my bum. Well, you do don't you? When she was three I decided to really try. I lost a lot of weight by eating sensibly and going to the gym with a personal trainer about four times a week.

I was fit for a while, but it required a lot of time and dedication. And then I got pregnant again. I was 36 when I had Cameron. I didn't put on as much weight this time but I was still a size 12ish and I didn't want to be. I wanted to be what I was when I was twenty, a size 8 to 10.

So three years ago I tried my first detox. A friend of mine had given it a go after being recommended to do so by Ko Chohan. I hadn't seen my friend in months but when I saw her again her skin was beautiful and she just looked well. So, I thought, why not? I turned to Ko and asked her what could this do for me and she explained what I needed to do. After a week on the detox I had a headache and didn't feel too good, but I kept to the plan (although I did wonder occasionally) for a month. By that time I'd lost a dress size, had so much energy I was even more irritating than I normally am and had altered the way I eat for ever.

Six months later I did it again and this time I stuck to it quite rigidly because I knew I would gain great results. I lost yet another dress size and felt better still. My cellulite had diminished dramatically and my skin was smoother than it had ever been. I felt alive. And remember, all this without counting calories or going to the gym.

The detox has given me a fantastic freedom because I just don't worry about weight any more. I'm in control now. I don't feel guilty about food and it's easy, because I'm doing what I want to do. And before you think I've turned into one of those boring Stepford Wives women who seem to find time to iron their knickers, I haven't. I can't spend hours cultivating the perfect courgette risotto. I know that you and I have a thousand things to do in a day. We have families to look after, careers to follow, offices to get to, shopping to do and somehow, in all of that, some sleep to catch up on. And that is why we need a plan that is completely practical, something that shows us what to do so that we don't have to think about it too much. Something that gives us energy and makes us feel good. That is why this book can work for you.

A couple of years ago, people started to ask me how I'd managed to lose so much weight. There was some publicity about it and the comments and questions came rolling in. Thousands of letters landed on my desk asking for more information. Some thought I'd been drinking magical green slime for three months and not eaten a thing.

Some thought I'd become bulimic. A couple of dieticians had a go at me because they thought I was starving myself, which wasn't true because I eat more food now, not less. There was a lot of misinformation and speculation, so I put a video together to explain it all. *Carol Vorderman's 28 Day Detox Diet* video became a best-seller and the response was phenomenal. Supermarkets claimed massive increases in the sale of vegetables and non-wheat food. Health food shops quickly ran out of supplements and foods that we'd recommended – so much so that they wanted advance warning of the publication date of this book.

Well, *The 28 Day Detox Diet* book took the shops by storm, and took all of us by surprise. In its first year of publication, half a million copies were sold and have been used successfully by men and women alike. Thousands and thousands of letters and emails have flooded in, many with personal stories from people who had followed the detox and were thrilled with it. I've been stopped in the street by men and women who are giggling with happiness with the results they've had. People who've lost stones in weight and feel younger and healthier than they have for years. Men who say that it has transformed the women in their lives, so they are now trying it for themselves.

But the questions never ended either. Many wanted to know how to continue eating once they'd finished the initial 28 days. Could we have more recipes? What other supplements should I take? Can I ever eat chocolate again? What should I eat in restaurants?

That is why this book covers both the 28 day detox as well as how to maintain healthy eating once that is over. In other words, *Detox for Life*. We've packed it with shopping lists, menu plans (which you can choose to follow if you want), recipes, advice and guidelines so that you can take advantage of all the health benefits that the detox offers. Not just while you're on it, but after the first 28 days as well. You see, after you've completed your first 28 days, you will definitely want to know more. You'll be conscious of exactly what kind of food you're eating for probably the first time in your life.

For instance, you'll be aware of different fats. On the detox we avoid dairy products and all the fats associated with them. You'll learn about the best fats to boost your system and give you energy, fats which are found naturally in certain foods and oils.

You will also notice the immediate effect eating things like cream cakes has on you. You'll find that you don't want to eat them, not because of calories, not because of any 'naughty but nice' guilt, but simply because you don't fancy it.

You will lose any wish to go back to any diets you tried before. Diets that have strict portion control or those that offer low-calorie alternatives to the real thing (which usually means you eat two 'low-calorie' biscuits instead of one normal one, making no difference whatsoever) will be a thing of the past. You will finally realise that it doesn't need to be that way.

I cannot stress enough that this is not about counting calories, it is not about guilt, it is not about eating less.

It is about eating more and it is about several positive things that you will find happening to your body. Your shape changes, your eyes sparkle, your skin glows, you sleep better, you take fewer medicines and you feel alive when you wake up in the mornings.

If you stick to the detox for 28 days and your body is well enough then this is what will happen to you:

You will feel alive and energetic

Your health will improve

You will lose weight

You will lose inches

Picture it now and think about it. You can do it. Give it a go. Go on.

CHAPTER 1

REAL SUCCESS

Carole Platten, 33, hairdresser

'My self-esteem had reached an all-time low. I was really unhappy about my weight and the way I looked. I always felt lacking in energy and suffered a lot from bloating. I had dieted plenty of times in the past but the weight never stayed off – I always went back to old ways, so was desperate to do something about my weight and my health.

Before I started the detox diet I must admit I ate a lot of junk foods. Because my job as a hairdresser doesn't allow for many breaks, I was in the habit of grabbing quick foods – chocolate, fizzy drinks, crisps, convenience meals – just to keep me going.

At first I found it hard to give up my cup of tea in the morning. I used to rely on it to get me going! I also missed my coffee, alcohol and chocolate to start with. But I substituted sugary snacks with healthy snacks such as nuts and seeds and found that my energy levels improved enormously. I no longer experienced energy highs and lows throughout the day. By week 3, I found that I needed less sleep yet would wake up in the morning feeling alert and raring to go. That was unheard of before!

Amazingly, I lost a whole stone. I was thrilled to have dropped from a size 16 to 14 after 28 days. My clothes almost hung off me!

But it wasn't just the weight loss that spurred me on. My skin became clearer and the condition of my hair really improved. I experienced less bloating once I gave up wheat and no longer craved all those sugary snacks.

As I felt so good, I continued to eat the same foods beyond the initial 28 days. I now eat healthily all the time, which doesn't mean that I can't indulge myself with the occasional pudding or chocolate if I really want to! I have learned to listen to my body rather than my head!

The biggest change for me was the improvement in my self-esteem. As a result of the detox diet, I feel so positive about myself. I love being able to wear skimpy clothes and feeling so well.'

Maureen Sansom, 56, deputy manager of a residential home

'I have a very stressful job which, in the past, made it difficult to stick to a healthy diet. I used to comfort eat as a way of unwinding when I got home. But, of course, that never actually solved anything and would only make me feel more tired and miserable. It was all too easy to reach for a chocolate bar rather than doing something energetic like going for a walk!

Before detoxing, I felt very tired all the time and had trouble sleeping. I knew that I had to change my ways if I wanted to feel better and cope better with my job. That's why I decided to try the detox diet.

The hardest thing for me was giving up coffee and dairy products. I depended on coffee to get me through the day so it was a big habit to break. I substituted herbal teas and dandelion root tea for coffee and quickly felt much better. I also loved cheese and, being vegetarian, was a bit worried about missing out on protein. However, once I cut out dairy products I found that the symptoms of my ulcerative colitis [an inflammation of the lower gut] eased noticeably. I included more nuts and seeds in my diet to make sure I got enough protein.

I took my own food with me to work – oatcakes, hummus, seeds and even my own wheat-free muesli for breakfast when I had an early start. My work colleagues and friends soon noticed how well I was looking. That really encouraged me.

During the 28 day detox diet I lost 12 pounds and went from a size 14 to a size 12. For the first time in my life, the weight has stayed off and has not yo-yoed up and down as it used to! My skin is much clearer and I look so much more awake. In fact I began sleeping much better after the second week on the detox diet. My old sleeping problems have completely disappeared.

I am no longer tired when I get home from work. I have a lot more energy and no longer want to comfort eat. What's more, I have found that I actually save money because I am not buying all those junk foods.'

Sarah Culhane, 42, mother of four children

'After all the excesses of Christmas I was left feeling sluggish and in desperate need of a kick-start. I had had my fill of rich food and alcohol. It was as if my body was telling me that enough was enough. I had gained excess fat, my clothes felt tighter, I felt bloated and, quite honestly, I wanted to get my body back into gear again.

The most difficult part of the detox diet was coping with cooking for the rest of the family. With four children and a husband to feed, I had very little time to cook for myself. So I coped by bulk cooking – big bowls of tomato, vegetable and lentil soups and chickpea and vegetable hot pots – so that I always had a meal for myself ready. I also adapted favourite recipes in line with the detox rules, to give me new ideas for meals. I used a lot of pulses in family meals too and, surprise, surprise, the kids loved them! In fact they got quite fond of lentils and risottos in the end!

I found I got headaches for the first few days. This was put down to giving up caffeine and alcohol – a bit of a shock to the system – but the headaches disappeared completely after day 4.

Giving up my near-continual consumption of Earl Grey tea was hard at first. I replaced it with water and herb tea. I would take my own supply of herb tea bags to social events to help me stick to the diet.

Children's teatime was always a danger time before I did the detox diet. I would be tempted to eat all the leftovers. So I made sure that I had a supply of healthy snacks such as fruit, brazil nuts, oatcakes, rye crispbreads and avocados to satisfy my hunger at that time of day.

I didn't intend to lose weight but was pleasantly surprised to have lost 8 pounds after 28 days – quite a bonus really, considering I never felt hungry! I had less bloat, my stomach became flatter, my thighs looked trimmer and my clothes fitted much better.

The biggest difference was the way I felt inside. I felt re-energised and ready to take on the daily routines again. It was as if my batteries had been recharged and I had a new spark of life.

Now I return to the detox diet whenever I feel in need of "purification". For example, if I've had a spate of socialising, eating too much rich food, drinking a little too much alcohol, then I detox for a few days. That rejuvenates my mind and body and puts me back on track.'

Emma Woollen, 35, nursery assistant

'I had been trying to lose weight on and off for several years but without any lasting success. I found most diets were too restrictive and left me feeling hungry, weak and frustrated. I had bought Carol's video, which I found inspirational, but then Carol Vorderman's Detox for Life gave me a realistic eating plan that I could fit into my lifestyle.

I followed the 28 day diet during April 2002, which overlapped with the school holidays and work. That meant that I had to be well organised, shopping with a list and preparing meals in advance. But I quickly learnt to fit my eating around family meals and adapted some of the recipes to suit the children. For them, I added a little meat or fish and increased the potatoes or rice.

I was surprised how much I enjoyed preparing and eating the meals. Unlike other diets, I didn't find the 28 day detox restrictive because there were plenty of delicious permitted snacks. I loved to snack on nuts and fresh fruit. For a treat I would eat fresh dates or strawberries. Even my children now eat more fruit!

I found the diet plan easy to follow because there was no calorie counting. I learnt to eat whenever I felt hungry and to stop when I was full. I even stopped craving chocolate – something that I had never imagined possible – because my body didn't want it. Mostly, I preferred fruit.

I always felt in control of my eating. I even ate out in my favourite Italian restaurant several times during the 28 day plan, choosing the healthier options on the menu, without anybody noticing that I was on a "diet".

The diet has made a big difference to the way I shop now. I supplement my weekly supermarket shopping with an extra trip or two to the local greengrocer. That means that I always have a good choice of interesting fruit and vegetables in the house and there's no excuse for a takeaway by the end of the week!

I lost 9 pounds on the 28 day detox diet, which is most noticeable around my stomach and hips. I went from a size 14 to size 12. Best of all, the weight has stayed off. I feel much healthier, I sleep better and I have a lot more energy than ever before.'

Sarah Lawes, 24, agricultural business consultant

'Around the end of 2001, I was feeling tired all the time and generally run down. My doctor ruled out any medical causes and simply put it down to the stresses of fast living. That's when I knew I had to take stock of my health and change my eating habits.

I had always been interested in detoxing, despite knowing very little about it, so when I saw Carol Vorderman's Detox For Life, I knew that this was the perfect opportunity to clean up my diet and improve my health. Carol is a great role model for me because she always looks so full of energy and years younger than her age.

I followed the detox diet with my friend/housemate. We took it in turns to cook and prepare food in the evenings. Not only did this help to keep us really motivated, but having to cook only on alternate days helped me to cope with my long working hours.

I prepared my lunches the day before and took them to work with me – soup in a flask, tubs of salad and, my absolute favourite, quinoa and rice pilaff. On cold days, when I didn't fancy salad, I would heat up my meal in a microwave at work. If I had to attend a business lunch, I simply chose the healthier options and kept to the diet plan the rest of the day. I often had to work longer hours so I kept my energy up by snacking on rice cakes, sultanas and nuts.

I stuck closely to the 28 day plan but did allow myself a tiny piece of dark chocolate daily. That was my one indulgence but it satisfied my chocolate craving.

The biggest benefit I gained from the detox diet was feeling healthy. Within just a few days, I no longer felt tired and I had heaps of energy – something I hadn't experienced for ages.

Weight loss was not my goal. Although I probably did drop a few pounds after 28 days, that was just a bonus compared with the way I felt. My stomach became a lot flatter once I cut out wheat, even though I didn't think that bloating was a particular issue for me before. I have continued to eat a wheat-free diet since completing the 28 day detox because I feel lighter and more comfortable. In fact, my diet has remained really healthy and, although I don't consciously detox, I regularly make many of the recipes in the detox diet. I have invested in a steamer, stopped buying ready-made sauces, and would rather snack on a handful of dried fruit and nuts than a biscuit.

After completing the 28 day detox I have grown to love delicious healthy food!'

CHAPTER 2
ALL ABOUT DETOXING

Why detox?

Do you feel lethargic, heavy and generally under the weather? Do your skin and hair look dull and lifeless? And have your energy levels reached rock bottom? If you are feeling all of these things, you will definitely benefit from this detox diet. Toxicity has got a habit of creeping up on you. Symptoms like achy joints, vague pains, tiredness, weight gain and headaches are easy to ignore most of the time. You probably put them down to the stresses of everyday living, or simply regard them as a natural part of the ageing process. But they are often early warning signs that your body isn't coping with toxins as well as it ought to.

Any stressful period can result in similar symptoms of toxin build-up, particularly when you let good eating, exercise and relaxation habits lapse and don't look after your body as well as you should do. Christmas is, of course, the classic time for over-indulging in rich food and alcohol. It's hardly surprising, then, that you end up feeling sluggish and bloated in the new year. Lack of sleep, stress, anxiety and lack of exercise all take their toll on your body. What's more, if you smoke, take regular medication or drink lots of coffee your poor body has an even bigger toxic load to deal with.

This is where the 28 day detox diet can help you. It will give your strained digestive system a rest by helping to eliminate the overload on your system and restore your natural energy levels. During the 28 day detox you will not only lose excess weight but you will quickly begin to feel healthier and happier.

Do you need to detox?

When your system becomes overburdened with toxins, you develop a pattern of symptoms. One or two symptoms are probably no cause for concern, but when you develop a number of symptoms, that's when you need to take stock. Complete the symptoms questionnaire on the right to find out whether you need to detox.

What will the detox diet do for you?

Detoxing will do wonders for the way you look, the way you feel and your ability to cope with stress. Like me, you may well find that you lose excess weight when you are detoxing because you will be eating healthier foods and feeling more positive about yourself. I dropped two dress sizes the first time I did the detox diet. But you should regard weight loss as more of a bonus than a major aim of the detox programme. It's a sign that your body is rebalancing and working well. Here's a quick rundown of the benefits you can expect during the detox diet.

Improved appearance

Your eyes will begin to look brighter, your skin will become clearer, the condition of your hair will improve and your nails will become stronger.

Inner calm

You will feel more relaxed and less stressed as your hormones become better balanced. You will find that you are able to think more clearly and remember things better – quite a plus really!

Better sleep

You will find that you sleep much better. If you have previously had difficulty in getting to sleep and staying asleep, this detox diet could transform your nights. And the best part is that you wake feeling refreshed and energised in the morning.

This questionnaire is not intended to diagnose or treat any illness or underlying medical condition. You should always check with your doctor if you suspect you may have an allergy, infection or medical condition.

❏ Do you find it increasingly hard to lose weight?
❏ Do you tend to gain weight readily?
❏ Do you have cellulite?
❏ Do you suffer from frequent headaches?
❏ Do you often feel fatigued and lethargic?
❏ Do you feel sluggish?
❏ Do you suffer from bloating?
❏ Do you suffer skin problems such as eczema, acne or psoriasis?

- ❑ Do you sometimes have joint and muscle aches?
- ❑ Do you feel run-down?
- ❑ Have you developed food intolerances (e.g. wheat or dairy) during adulthood?
- ❑ Do you suffer from constipation, diarrhoea or irritable bowel syndrome?
- ❑ Do you suffer from recurrent colds and minor infections?
- ❑ Do you have mood swings?
- ❑ Are you often irritable or restless?
- ❑ Do you suffer from indigestion or heartburn?

If you ticked eight or more boxes you definitely need to detox.

If you ticked between four and eight boxes you are beginning to show signs of toxicity and may benefit from a detox programme.

If you ticked fewer than four boxes you are unlikely to have a toxicity problem but you will still benefit to maintain good health.

Good health

Detoxing brings numerous health benefits. It will boost your immune system – you'll be far less susceptible to colds and minor infections – and allow your liver, kidneys and bowels to work more efficiently. In the long term, you greatly reduce your risk of chronic diseases such as heart disease, diabetes, cancer and arthritis.

What is detoxing?

Detoxing is the way your body gets rid of potentially harmful chemicals (toxins). It's a process that goes on all the time, thanks to your body's processing machinery, or detoxifiers (see below). In fact, your body is designed to cope with toxins. The problem arises when you take in more toxins than your body can handle, or your body's detoxifiers cannot carry out their job quite as well as they should. Your system becomes overloaded and you develop all sorts of symptoms including bloating, lack of energy and dull skin. That's when you need to give your body a helping hand: when it's time to embark on the detox diet.

What are toxins?

Toxins are substances that are capable of harming your body. These substances can be naturally produced in the body (like carbon dioxide) or they can enter your body from the air you breathe, the food and drink you consume or as chemicals absorbed through your skin. In fact, you probably don't realise that you are bombarded by toxins every day. These come from pollutants in the air, cigarette smoke, exhaust fumes, detergents, household chemicals and toxic metals in the environment such as mercury and lead. And then there's the cocktail of pesticide residues and artificial additives in your food as well as the toxins found in alcohol, caffeine, drugs and medications.

Your body's own detoxifiers

The liver, kidneys, gut, skin and lungs are the organs most involved in ridding your body of harmful substances and waste products. Here's a quick guide to how they handle toxins.

Liver

This is your body's main processing plant. Its job is to make safe – detoxify – all potentially harmful substances. Once disarmed, these substances can then be eliminated via the kidneys, lungs or bowel. This work is carried out by thousands of enzymes. These enzymes require certain nutrients to help them to do their job. This is where your diet can really help your liver.

Foods to help your liver
Cruciferous vegetables (Brussels sprouts, broccoli, cabbage, cauliflower); sulphur-containing foods (onions, garlic); brightly coloured fruit and vegetables (tomatoes, apricots, peppers, blueberries, carrots); lemons.

Supplements to help your liver
Milk thistle, artichoke extract, garlic, dandelion, fennel.

Kidneys

Their job is to filter out waste products such as urea (which is produced when the body breaks down proteins) from your blood into your urine. It's amazing to think that 7 litres (12 pints) of fluid pass through your kidneys every hour, so it's important to drink plenty of water to dilute the toxins and to help the kidneys carry out their job efficiently.

Foods to help your kidneys
Water; all fruit and vegetables; parsley leaf; herbal teas.

Supplements to help your kidneys
Dandelion; horsetail; goldenrod; cranberry; celery seed.

Gut

Your intestines not only process nutrients and toxins, but also propel indigestible material such as fibre, and potential toxins (from the bile) to the bowel. Fibre helps to mop up some of the toxins, stopping them getting absorbed into your body and carrying them to the bowel. Here they are disarmed by friendly bacteria and eliminated in the faeces.

Foods to help your gut
Fibre-rich foods: fruit (especially apples, prunes, berries, dried fruit); vegetables (especially carrots, broccoli, cabbage); flaxseeds (linseeds); beans; lentils; oats (unless you are gluten intolerant); barley.

Supplements to help your gut
Fibre supplements (psyllium); probiotic supplements; fructo-oligosaccharides; aloe vera; chlorella.

Skin

This plays a big role in getting rid of toxins. Some toxins are eliminated in your sweat, others in your skin oils (sebum) and others via the shedding of dead skin cells.

Foods to help your skin
Water; fruit and vegetables; flaxseeds; essential oils (flax oil, walnut oil, pumpkinseed oil or blended essential oils); pumpkinseeds.

Supplements to help your skin
Ginkgo biloba; essential fatty acid supplements (flaxseed oil, evening primrose oil); antioxidant supplements; golden seal root.

Lymphatic circulation

This is like a drainage system. It carries waste products and potential toxins that are too large to enter your bloodstream from your cells to the lymph nodes for processing. They are then returned to the bloodstream and are finally delivered to the liver for detoxification.

Foods and herbs to help your lymphatic circulation
Water; echinacea; sarsaparilla root.

Other ways to help your lymphatic circulation
Manual lymphatic drainage massage; dry skin brushing; Epsom bath salts.

Lungs

They filter out waste gases that you produce in your body, such as carbon dioxide, as well as toxic gases that you breathe in.

Foods to help your lungs
Fruit and vegetables (especially apples, onions, blueberries, blackberries and raspberries).

Supplements to help your lungs
Antioxidant supplements.

How does the detox diet work?

The aim of this detox diet is to give your body a break from its usual toxin load by reducing the amount of toxins you take in and encouraging your body to eliminate old toxins. More specifically, it involves the following.

- Eating the right food to encourage the body's natural detoxification processes.
- Going organic wherever possible (don't worry if you cannot always eat organic produce – eating the right types of food is more important).
- Cutting out addictive toxic substances such as nicotine, caffeine and alcohol.
- Cutting down on foods and drinks that add to your toxin load – processed sugars, saturated fats, salty foods and additives.
- Including certain supplements and herbs that support liver function and help detoxification.
- Reducing emotional and physical stress in your life.
- Adopting healthy habits such as exercise, relaxation therapies and complementary therapies.

Remember

Don't feel you need to make all of these changes at the same time. Make gradual changes to suit your lifestyle. These will become habits of a lifetime rather than quick fixes that don't last.

Check with your doctor

Before starting this or any other detox diet programme you should consult your doctor, in particular with regard to any allergies you have to any of the foods, drinks, products, supplements or other recommendations contained in this programme. This detox diet may not be suitable for everyone. Pregnant women should be especially careful and ensure that their doctor advises that the detox diet is suitable for them. If you are taking any medication or have any medical condition, you should check with your doctor first.

CHAPTER 3
SIMPLE PRINCIPLES OF THE DETOX DIET

Do not weigh yourself

The main aim of this detox diet is not to lose weight! Of course, you may well lose excess pounds, but this should not be your main focus. Concentrate instead on how much energy you have, how well you sleep and how good you feel physically and mentally.

Don't be tempted to jump on the scales every day. Even if your clothes feel looser and you can finally get into those jeans, it is important to resist the temptation to find out how much you weigh. That number on the scales is not important. What matters is how much better you will feel.

Do not count calories

Unlike other diets, which are designed for weight loss and little else, this detox diet does not require you to count calories. In fact, you are not expected to count or weigh anything! What this detox diet teaches you is to eat sensibly, so that eventually you will instinctively know how much to eat and what is right for your body. Listen to your body and tune into how your body feels.

Never go hungry

On the detox diet you should never go hungry or miss meals. This is not a starvation diet. Eat when you are hungry. Sounds too good to be true? Well, it really works, because the foods included in this diet – fruit, vegetables, whole grains and pulses – are filling and satisfying. They are packed with fibre and water and send a powerful signal to your brain that your appetite has been satisfied, so any desire to keep on eating and eating goes away.

The main reason many people overeat is because they follow diets that confuse the body's natural appetite control. Highly processed foods such as buns, crisps, cakes, biscuits, chocolate, ready meals and sauces are jam-packed with calories but lacking in fibre, nutrients and water. Without these important elements, your appetite cannot easily be satisfied because your brain will not receive that 'full' signal during your meal. That's why it's so easy to overeat these foods without feeling full. This detox diet aims to put you back in control of your appetite by eliminating the 'junk' element of the food you eat.

Drink water or herbal teas

Drinking plenty of fluid is absolutely vital while you are detoxing as it helps to eliminate water-soluble toxins from your body. It also helps to prevent constipation, reduce bloating and encourage clear skin.

Drink 6 to 8 glasses of water each day (between 1½ and 2 litres), although you will need more in hot weather or on days when you are exercising. As a rule of thumb, aim to drink an extra half litre of water for every hour you exercise. Choose still mineral water, or tap water that has been filtered, or boiled and then cooled. Ideally drink water that is at room temperature.

If you don't always fancy water, herbal teas – preferably loose leaf rather than tea bags – are excellent alternatives. Peppermint, camomile, dandelion root, horsetail and yarrow are particularly good as their essential oils help the detox process. Rooibosch tea is also beneficial as it is rich in antioxidants.

Fitting in 6 to 8 glasses of liquid a day isn't difficult once you get into the habit. Have a glass of water with a little freshly squeezed lemon juice or root ginger when you wake up – this is great for kick-starting your digestive system and bowel – then aim to drink little and often throughout the day. Have a glass before each meal, a glass between meals, another during the evening and perhaps a final glass of water last thing at night. Remember, some of these glasses can actually be herbal teas or freshly squeezed juices.

Eat foods as close to their natural state as possible

This means choosing fresh food whenever possible and eating most of your fruit and vegetables raw, for example as snacks, crudités, salads and juices. Raw food is full of vital nutrients, phytochemicals and enzymes. Once food has been kept too long, or if it has been cooked or processed in any way, its nutritional value plummets. Here are some tips on getting the most nutrition from your food.

- Make at least half of your diet raw fruit, vegetables, nuts and seeds.
- Buy fruit and vegetables in season whenever possible.
- Shop little and often – don't stock up.
- Buy locally grown produce if you can, ideally from farm shops and local markets.
- Buy British if you have a choice – imported produce is usually harvested underripe (before it has developed its full vitamin quota) and will have lost much of its nutritional value during its journey to your supermarket.
- Buy fresh-looking, unblemished, undamaged fruit and vegetables.
- Do not buy fresh produce that is nearing its sell-by date.
- Buy loose and not pre-packaged where possible.

Choose organic food where possible

You do not need to switch to a totally organic diet on this detox diet, especially as the cost can be very high, but selecting just a few organic ingredients will be a step in the right direction. If you can't buy many organic foods, don't worry. It's more important that you eat plentiful amounts of fresh foods – even if they are non-organic – than skimp on quantities. However, there are three main reasons for going organic on this detox diet.

- Organic foods are produced without the use of artificial pesticides and fertilisers, so they contain the lowest possible amounts of artificial, potentially toxic chemicals (such as nitrates). Although it's a controversial area, there is evidence that the 'cocktail' effect of pesticide residues over time may cause health problems in the future.
- Organic foods undergo minimal processing. That means they contain no hydrogenated fats, artificial additives, preservatives or genetically modified organisms (GMOs).
- Certain organic foods taste better and have more flavour.

- Buy fruit and vegetables in season when they are cheaper.
- Buy at least one organic variety of fruit or vegetable in your weekly shopping.
- Start with apples, potatoes, carrots, tomatoes and salad leaves.
- Join a local box scheme or visit a farmer's market – they offer the best value.
- Snap up seasonal offers or promotions.

Take detox supplements

While on the detox diet, you should take the following supplements to help support your liver and aid the whole detox process. More details about what each supplement does and how much to take are given in Chapter 8: Nutrition and Supplement Guide (see page 203). You will benefit from all six supplements but if you wish to try a deeper cleanse you may add other herbal supplements to your programme. In this case it is best to seek the advice of a qualified nutritional practitioner.

- Antioxidant supplement
- Milk thistle
- Kelp
- Essential oil blend (cold pressed seed oil consisting of omega 3 and 6)
- Spirulina
- Chlorella

What to eat

Fruit and vegetables

All types can be included but make sure you eat a broad range of them each day. That way you will get a better mix of the important phytochemicals (beneficial plant substances). Each day aim to eat at least three portions of fruit. Mix colours – yellow, orange, red – so you get a good balance of vitamins and antioxidants (see Chapter 8: Nutrition and Supplement Guide, pages 203–14).

Have fruit for desserts, for snacks in between meals or as freshly squeezed juices and smoothies (see pages 137–41 for recipes). Dried fruit may be included in small quantities. Have at least three portions of vegetables daily. All varieties of vegetables are good for detoxifying. Make at least one of these a cruciferous vegetable (broccoli, Brussels sprouts, cabbage, watercress or cauliflower) as these contain glucosinolates, which boost the activity of your liver's detoxifying enzymes. Vegetables are best eaten raw in salads or lightly steamed to get the most nutrients from them. You can also use them for juicing (see recipes on pages 137–41).

The most beneficial fruits and vegetables on a detox diet include those given in the shopping list (see Chapter 4, page 40).

Grains, bread and pasta

Take a break from wheat and try different types of whole grains, bread and pasta (see What to avoid, page 25). Millet, brown rice, quinoa, buckwheat, wheat-free and yeast-free bread, 100 per cent rye bread, pumpernickel bread, rye crackers, oatcakes, rice cakes and wheat-free pasta are all suitable. Oats contain smaller amounts of gluten than wheat and may be included but are best avoided if you are prone to bloating or you have a gluten sensitivity.

Whole grains provide fibre, vitamins (such as the B vitamins and vitamin E), minerals (such as potassium, magnesium, zinc, iron and selenium), complex carbohydrate and small amounts of essential oils. These foods, along with most fruits and vegetables, provide slow-releasing carbohydrates, which provide more sustained energy.

Aim to include one portion of grains, bread or pasta in each meal. See the shopping list (Chapter 4, page 40) for suitable varieties.

Pulses and sprouted beans

Pulses provide protein as well as B vitamins, iron, zinc and fibre. Ideally, buy dried pulses, soak and cook according to the instructions on the packet. Tinned pulses are a useful stand-by but make sure you drain them and wash them well if they have been canned in salty water. You can include any variety of beans, lentils and bean sprouts on the detox diet. The different varieties are given under the shopping list (see Chapter 4, page 41). Sprouted beans are excellent on a detox diet. They are rich in valuable enzymes, vitamins and minerals as well as protein. You can buy them from health food stores or supermarkets. Alternatively, you can grow your own sprouts.

Mung beans, chickpeas, aduki beans and alfalfa seeds are all suitable for sprouting. Simply soak about a tablespoon in water overnight. Drain and rinse, then put them in a sprouting jar or a wide-necked glass jar (see Checklist of essentials, page 30). Rinse them daily until they start to sprout. They are ready to eat when the shoots are about 1 cm high.

Cold-pressed oils

Cold-pressed seed and nut oils, such as flaxseed, pumpkinseed, walnut, sesame and sunflower, can all be included. Pumpkinseed, flaxseed and walnut are rich in omega-3 oils, while sesame and sunflower oils are rich in omega-6 oils. You need to get the right balance of these oils each day (see Chapter 8: Nutrition and Supplement Guide, page 204), which is why you may find a seed oil blend easier. It takes much of the guesswork out! Aim to have between 1 and 4 tablespoons per day, or a little less if you include seeds and nuts as well.

Like nuts and seeds, the nutritional value of these oils is easily destroyed by heating and by exposure to light and air. So store them in dark bottles in a cool dark place. Don't use them for frying. Instead, use them in dressings or for drizzling over baked potatoes and steamed vegetables.

Nuts and seeds

All kinds of nuts and seeds can be included in the detox diet, although almonds, brazils and cashew nuts are the most beneficial. Check the shopping list (Chapter 4, page 41). Nuts and seeds are rich in essential fats, the omega-3 and omega-6 oils (see Chapter 8: Nutrition and Supplement Guide, page 204), protein, fibre, vitamins and minerals. Far from being fattening, they are packed with important nutrients that help detoxification, benefit your health and reduce many of the symptoms of ageing and ill health.

Choose plain, unsalted nuts and avoid those with coatings or flavourings. Lightly toast nuts and seeds under a grill or in a hot oven for a few minutes. This will bring out their wonderful nutty flavour.

To get the right intake of essential fats, you need to eat around 1 heaped tablespoon of nuts or seeds a day. Since you need both omega-3 and omega-6 oils, you should include some flaxseeds (linseeds) or pumpkinseeds each day. Since flaxseeds are quite hard, you will get more nutrients from them by grinding them in a coffee grinder and then sprinkling them on salads, muesli or stews. You can even stir them into fruit smoothies.

Essential fats are easily oxidised (damaged) and lose their nutritional value if exposed to the air, or if they are heated or stored for too long. So store them in an airtight jar, in a cool, dark place. Also, check the best before date on the packet to make sure they are as fresh as possible.

Non-dairy milk

Almond, sesame and rice milks are all suitable for you to use while you are detoxifying. They do, of course, taste a little different from cow's milk, but you will quickly get used to the taste. You can use them in exactly the same way as you would do cow's milk – on muesli, in porridge, or as a drink. You can make your own almond milk by soaking a handful of blanched almonds overnight in 300 ml of water (use a little more water if you prefer a thinner milk). Remove the skins then whiz in a blender, with an optional vanilla pod for additional flavour, until smooth.

Soya milk and other soya products are best kept to a minimum. If you do include it, go for organic, unsweetened soya milk.

Fresh herbs, spices, flavouring

Fresh herbs (such as coriander, basil, oregano, mint, parsley, marjoram), spices, lemon juice, lime juice, freshly ground black pepper and cider vinegar can all be used to add flavour to cooked dishes and salads in place of salt. In fact fresh herbs are particularly beneficial on a detox diet. Most varieties help digestion and have a natural cleansing effect. Spices, such as ginger, coriander seeds, dill, caraway and fennel seeds are really useful because they also help digestion. See the shopping list (Chapter 4, page 41).

What to avoid

Wheat products

Try to avoid wheat altogether while you are on the detox diet. Wheat contains gluten, a protein that many people find hard to digest and which can cause bloating and wind. This mild sensitivity is fairly common, and you may not realise you have it until you omit wheat from your diet. On the detox diet, by excluding wheat you will find that these symptoms will improve. You may be able to reintroduce certain wheat products after 28 days and thereafter eat them in moderation. However, those with a true gluten allergy – a condition called coeliac disease – must avoid all sources of gluten for life.

The most common wheat products to avoid while you are detoxifying include the following:

- Bread
- Wheat-based breakfast cereals
- Ordinary (durum wheat) pasta
- White, brown and wholemeal (wheat) flour
- Ordinary (wheat) noodles
- Couscous
- Cakes
- Biscuits

Caffeine

Caffeine is a stimulant that mimics the effects of stress on the body and depletes it of essential nutrients. Coffee, tea and caffeine-based soft drinks are often used as a quick fix to boost flagging energy levels and concentration by making you feel more alert. But the effect is short-lived. Drinking several cups of coffee throughout the day can leave you feeling more tired, irritable, restless and with a headache.

Cutting out Caffeine

If you have been used to drinking six or more cups of coffee or tea a day, don't give up overnight. This could lead to withdrawal symptoms, similar to caffeine toxicity, with headaches and irritability. Cut down on caffeine drinks gradually, over a period of a week or two, and replace them with water or herbal tea.

Alcohol

Alcohol should definitely be given a wide berth while you are detoxifying. The reason is that alcohol is a cell toxin. In the liver, alcohol is broken down to acetaldehyde – a toxin – which harms liver cells, the brain and muscles. It increases free radical production and destroys and uses up B vitamins and vitamins C and E. Alcohol acts like a diuretic, making your kidneys excrete more fluid as well as vital minerals such as magnesium, calcium and potassium.

Salt

Do not add salt to any foods during cooking or at the table. Instead, flavour your food with spices, freshly ground black pepper, fresh herbs, lemon and lime juice, or cider vinegar. You should avoid all processed food that contains salt. These include crisps, salted snacks, ready meals, ready-made sauces, condiments, stock cubes, breakfast cereals, soups and foods canned in brine. You get enough sodium (salt) from foods in their natural state. Fruit, vegetables and grains contain potassium, which helps to rebalance the sodium in your body and to flush out excess salt. High salt intakes can cause fluid retention, bloating and dehydration. Over a period of time, excess salt can increase the risk of high blood pressure in people who are susceptible.

Dairy products

Try to avoid dairy products on the detox diet. This includes milk, cheese, yoghurt, cream and butter. Many people find dairy products difficult to digest because of the lactose (milk sugar) content. This can cause bloating, discomfort and flatulence.

Dairy products can often create excess mucus in the sinuses and nasal passages. So having a break from dairy products may help reduce symptoms such as a persistent stuffy or runny nose, or congested sinuses. A little organic goat's or sheep's milk products may be tolerated but it is best to reintroduce these foods after you have completed the 28 day detox diet.

Meat and fish

Meat and fish are best avoided on the detox diet. That's because they create added work for your digestive system. Cutting them out encourages any old mucoid build-up in the gut to pass out and helps your gut regain its normal healthy functioning.

Processed food with artificial additives

Most ready meals, biscuits, cakes, desserts and spreads contain artificial additives (such as artificial sweeteners, colours, flavourings and preservatives), which may accumulate and produce harmful effects in your body in the long term. Any food containing additives should be avoided during the detox programme.

What to eat checklist

- Fresh fruit (limit bananas to 1 every other day)
- Vegetables (limit potatoes to 1 portion every 2 to 3 days)
- Salads
- Grains – millet, brown rice, quinoa, rye, buckwheat
- Breads – rye, wheat-free, pumpernickel
- Crispbreads – rye, rice cakes, oatcakes
- Water and herbal teas
- Freshly squeezed juices (carrot, apple, celery)
- Pulses and bean sprouts
- Rice, almond and sesame milk
- Nuts (brazil, almond, cashew)
- Seeds (sunflower, sesame, pumpkin, flax)
- Cold-pressed oils
- Fresh herbs

What to avoid checklist

- Coffee, tea and other caffeine drinks (including decaffeinated drinks)
- Dairy products – milk, cheese, yoghurt, cream
- Sugar
- Cakes, biscuits, confectionery
- Meat
- Fish
- Eggs
- Wheat bread, pasta, noodles, crackers
- White rice
- Ready meals
- Salt
- Alcohol
- Artificial food additives
- Fried foods
- Artificial sweeteners
- Hydrogenated fats
- Fizzy drinks
- Squashes and cordials

Coping without wheat

Instead of...	Eat
Wheat bread	Rye bread, pumpernickel bread and wheat-free bread
Wheat pasta	Pasta made from corn, quinoa, rice or millet
Wheat noodles	Soba (buckwheat) noodles and rice noodles
Wheat breakfast cereals	Muesli made from oat flakes, rye flakes or millet flakes and porridge made with oats or millet

Coping without dairy products

Instead of...	Eat
Milk	Rice, almond or sesame milk
Butter	Hummus, tahini, nut butter and guacamole

Coping without sugar

Instead of...	Eat
Cakes and biscuits	Fresh fruit
Sugary breakfast cereals	Muesli made from oat flakes, rye flakes or millet flakes and porridge made with oats or millet
Chocolate	Liquorice bars, fruit bars or sesame snaps for a treat
Confectionery	Raisins, sultanas, apricots, dates or marzipan balls (see recipe, page 75) for a treat
Squash, cordial	Freshly squeezed juices and water

Detox superfoods

Apples

Apples are very cleansing for the digestive system, encouraging the removal of toxins through the gut. They are rich in quercetin, a powerful antioxidant that has anti-cancer and anti-inflammatory actions. Eat apples unpeeled, as the quercetin is concentrated near and within the skin. Have apples as snacks, in fruit salads, grated on to cereal or as freshly squeezed juice.

Carrots

Carrots are terrific cleansers and are great for the skin, too. Rich in beta-carotene, a powerful antioxidant, they can help protect against lung cancer. The beta-carotene is best absorbed when eaten with a little fat or oil, or when eaten as part of a dressed salad, in stir-fries and casseroles or when juiced.

Garlic

The phytochemicals in garlic can help protect against heart disease, high blood pressure and colon cancer, and can also reduce blood cholesterol levels. It is a natural decongestant and its anti-viral, anti-bacterial properties help fight colds and infections. Crush garlic before adding it to dishes to release its beneficial compounds.

Broccoli

Broccoli and other cruciferous vegetables (Brussels sprouts, cauliflower and cabbage) are packed with beneficial phytochemicals that help fight cancer, especially of the bowel, stomach, breast, lungs and kidney. They are also rich in vitamin C, folic acid, calcium and beta-carotene. Eat raw in salads or as crudités, or steam briefly to conserve the nutrients.

Sprouted mung beans

Sprouted mung beans contain several times more vitamin C than unsprouted beans, as well as enzymes, protein and fibre. Eat them raw in salads or as a snack.

Lemons

Lemons have a strong cleansing effect and help stimulate the digestive system. They are full of vitamin C and are a great source of phytochemicals with well-known anti-cancer effects. The phytochemicals are found in the peel, pith and juice, so make use of the whole lemon. Use the peel to add zest to fruit salads and rice and quinoa salads. Use the juice in dressings or added to water for a refreshing and cleansing drink.

Quinoa

This nutty-flavoured tiny grain is rich in fibre, iron, magnesium and several B vitamins. Steam or boil and eat instead of pasta or rice or as a breakfast cereal. Mix into soups, pilafs and salads.

Papaya

Papayas contain vitamin C, beta-carotene, fibre and phytochemicals with strong antioxidant properties. They also contain a useful enzyme, papain, to help digestion. Use papayas in fruit salads or as a topping for muesli. They are also delicious in smoothies.

Flaxseeds (linseeds)

Flaxseeds (linseeds) are rich in heart-healthy omega-3 oils and contain the perfect natural fibre that protects your gut lining and prevents the absorption of bile acids. They help eliminate waste from the body, prevent constipation and encourage regular bowel movements. Choose pre-cracked organic golden flaxseeds (linseeds) and store in the fridge. Sprinkle on muesli, salads and porridge or use as a dessert topping.

CHAPTER 4
TIME FOR ACTION

When should you start the detox diet?

Of course, it is important that you choose the right time to start this detox diet. The time needs to feel right for you and you need to approach the detox diet with a positive frame of mind. The new year is often a good time to embark on a detox diet.

After the excesses of Christmas, your body will be in need of cleansing and will be ready to revitalise. This time of year is always a good time for decisions and renewed resolve! You may prefer to begin your detox diet in the spring. After all, this is the season of fresh starts and uplifted spirits. It is also the time of year when there is a greater choice of fruit and vegetables.

On the other hand, you may find it more motivating to embark on this detox diet a month or so before a holiday or special occasion. There's nothing like a big incentive to spur you on. The most important thing is to begin the 28 day detox diet with a positive attitude.

Get Support

It's also a good idea to enlist the support of your family or friends – people close to you. Tell them why you are doing the programme and how you are feeling. Let them know about the positive results you get but also call upon their encouragement if you have a 'down' day. Everyone hits little sticking points and that's when you need family and friends around to help pick you up again. You may even find that they want to join in your detox programme (see Chapter 7: Detox and Beyond, Family meals, page 201).

Checklist of essentials

You don't have to invest in expensive gadgets but the following kitchen items will help you to prepare your meals more easily.

- Steamer – excellent for lightly cooking your vegetables with minimum loss of valuable nutrients and flavour.
- Storage jars – keep dried foods such as beans, lentils, nuts and seeds in airtight storage jars and use them within six months.
- Blender – use either a hand blender or liquidiser for making soups and smoothies.
- Glass jars or sprouting jars – for sprouting mung beans, aduki beans, chickpeas, alfalfa, lentils, pumpkinseeds and sunflower seeds.
- Food processor – makes chopping and grating vegetables much easier for making soups, hot pots, stews and salads.
- Juicer – a bit of a luxury item but well worth the investment if your budget can stretch that far. See pages 138–41 for some delicious juice recipes.

Time for Change

The 28 day detox should be an enjoyable experience. During this time you will need to make a number of changes to your old eating habits. You will probably find that you eat different types or amounts of certain foods. You may eat foods in different combinations from those you are used to. You will have to make changes to your usual shopping habits and perhaps the way you prepare and cook meals. That's why it's important to start the detox diet when the time is right for you and you know you can commit to change.

How to prepare your food

Preparing and cooking food is very simple on this detox diet. Most of the dishes in the menu plans can be assembled in less than twenty minutes. You don't need great cooking skills either, just a bit of common sense and plenty of fresh ingredients to hand! Here are some useful tips to follow.

- Do not buy ready-cut vegetables, salads or fruit. They will have lost most of their nutritional value by the time you eat them.
- Prepare fruit and vegetables just before you make them into a salad or cook them. Once they are chopped they start to lose nutrients.
- Do not cook food too far in advance or reheat leftovers.

- Fruit and vegetables should be eaten unpeeled whenever possible because many vitamins and minerals are concentrated just beneath the skin.
- Use frozen food if fresh is not available – its nutritional value is similar.

How to cook your food

Try to eat as much of your food as close to its natural state as possible. Raw fruit and vegetables are best but, if you use the right cooking methods, you can retain most of the nutritional benefits. Here are a few tips.

Steaming

Steaming is by far the best way of cooking your vegetables. As the vegetables are not in contact with the cooking water, there is very little loss of vitamins. For example, broccoli can lose more than 60 per cent of its vitamin C when it is boiled but only 20 per cent when steamed. You can steam any vegetable, even root vegetables such as potatoes and carrots. Make sure the steamer fits your pan properly and that the level of the water is below the bottom of the steamer.

Boiling

If you must boil vegetables, use as little water as possible, boil the water before adding the vegetables and cook them for the minimum time. Drain them straight away and never leave to soak in the cooking water. Always use a lid to stop steam escaping.

Obviously you will need to boil soups and stews but this is fine because the cooking liquid is retained along with the nutrients.

Stir-frying

Stir-frying is also a good cooking method as the food is cooked very briefly and so retains most of its nutrients. On the detox diet, try to stir-fry in a small quantity of stock or water rather than oil. This is because the high temperatures change the chemical structure of most oils, making them potentially harmful for your body. Do add oil once removed from heat.

What else can you do?

To get the most out of the detox diet, you should consider making positive changes for your mind, body and spirit. Good health depends on a good balance between your physical, emotional, mental and spiritual health. If one element is lacking then it has a knock-on effect on the others and your body is not in harmony.

Exercise

There are numerous good reasons to get active.

- Faster fat loss.
- Increased metabolism.
- Greater sense of well-being.
- Higher sense of self-esteem.
- Reduced stress.
- More efficient removal of toxins.
- Better functioning of digestive system (including the bowel).
- Stronger bones.
- Healthier-looking skin and hair.

Most experts recommend thirty minutes of gentle or moderate exercise five days a week (or twenty minutes of hard exercise three times a week) but on the detox programme you should listen to your body and do what you can manage, particularly if you have not done any formal exercise for a while. Little and often is better than a couple of hard sessions a month. It's important that you enjoy your chosen activities and don't regard them as a chore. You need to be able to fit them easily into your daily routine otherwise you simply won't keep them up. Try Pilates, yoga, walking, stretching and swimming on the detox programme. You can add other activities as you become accustomed to regular exercise.

Dry skin brushing

It's amazing to think that your body gets rid of around ½kg (1lb) of waste products through your skin each day. That's why it's so important to look after your skin. If your pores get clogged with dead skin cells, the impurities will remain in your body, placing undue stress on your liver and kidneys and leading eventually to an overloaded system.

That's why daily dry skin brushing is so important on this detox programme. It keeps your pores clear, allows the skin to 'breathe', makes your skin look brighter and feel softer. Brushing also stimulates your blood flow and lymph flow, leading to more efficient removal of waste products.

So how do you do it? First, invest in a natural bristle brush or loofah. Start brushing at the soles of your feet, working up your legs, front, chest, back and finally your hands and arms. Avoid your face. Use firm, long strokes – really as firm as you can bear, brushing towards your heart to encourage blood flow. The whole process should take about 5 minutes – you'll feel quite warm afterwards because you will have stimulated your circulation.

Deep breathing and relaxation

The way you breathe affects the balance of your body and mind. If you are tense or stressed your breathing tends to be shallow. This means that you will take in less oxygen and it will be harder for your lungs to expel waste products and toxins. If you breathe deeply you will take in more oxygen, feel more relaxed and improve your overall health. Sounds obvious, really, but it's surprising how many of us don't get it right!

This is what you should do. Breathe in slowly through your nose, allowing your diaphragm to expand downwards. You'll be able to feel your abdomen rise. Pause for a moment then breathe out through your mouth.

Manual lymphatic drainage massage

There's nothing quite like a great massage, is there? All types of massage are beneficial for stimulating the circulation, but lymphatic drainage massage focuses on stimulating the lymphatic circulation (your body's drainage system that carries nutrients into cells and removes waste products). It's a gentle massage that encourages the removal of released toxins and leaves you with a wonderful feeling of relaxation. Soaking in Epsom salt baths, saunas and steam rooms before this will relax the muscles and encourage further elimination of toxins.

Complementary therapies

If you can afford it, treat yourself to at least one complementary treatment during the 28 day detox diet. Choose from reflexology, Indian head massage, reiki massage or the Alexander technique. Complementary therapies are very useful for rebalancing your physical, emotional, mental and spiritual state during your detox programme. You'll find yourself with a heightened sense of wellbeing and relaxation.

Shopping list

To help get your 28 day detox diet off to a super-healthy start, here is a ready-made shopping list containing all the permitted foods and drinks. Use it as the basis for developing your own weekly shopping list. Of course, you are not expected to buy every item, just choose the ones that appeal to you most. Buy seasonal fruit and vegetables for best value.

DRINKS

Mineral water (still)
Herbal teas (preferably loose leaf), such as:

peppermint, camomile, dandelion root, horsetail and yarrow

Rooibosch tea

NON-DAIRY MILK

Almond milk

Rice milk

Sesame milk

FRUIT

Apples
Apricots
Peaches
Papayas
Bananas
Cherries
Plums

Kiwi fruits
Blueberries
Strawberries
Raspberries
Blackberries
Melons
Mangoes

Pears
Grapefruits
Lemons
Limes
Satsumas
Clementines

VEGETABLES

Alfalfa
Artichokes
Asparagus
Avocado
Celery
Lettuce
Watercress
Green beans, runner beans

Spinach
Peas
Mangetout
Broccoli
Brussels sprouts
Cauliflower
Rocket
Potatoes
Sweet potatoes

Yams
Pumpkins
Peppers
Squashes
Courgettes
Onions
Garlic

GRAINS The following can be bought as whole grains, flakes (good for making 'porridge') or flour.

Millet
Brown rice
Quinoa
Buckwheat
Oats (avoid if you are

prone to bloating or if you have a gluten sensitivity)
Non-wheat pasta (e.g. corn, rice, millet)

PULSES AND BEANSPROUTS

Sprouted beans (e.g. mung, alfalfa, chickpeas)
Red kidney beans
Chickpeas
Black-eyed beans
Haricot beans
Butter beans
Lentils (red, green, brown)
Hummus

NUTS AND SEEDS

Almonds
Brazils
Walnuts
Pecans
Cashew
Hazelnuts
Pine nuts
Peanuts
Pumpkinseeds
Flaxseeds (linseeds)
Sesame seeds
Sunflower seeds

BREADS AND CRISPBREADS

Wheat-free yeast-free bread
100 per cent rye bread
Pumpernickel bread
Rye crackers
Oatcakes
Rice cakes

COLD-PRESSED OILS

Essential oil blend
Flaxseed
Pumpkinseed
Walnut
Sesame
Sunflower
Extra-virgin olive oil

GRAINS Selection of fresh herbs (otherwise dried)

Coriander
Mint
Chives
Parsley
Basil
Marjoram
Oregano
Dill

SPICES

Cumin seeds and ground cumin
Cardamom
Ginger
Coriander seeds and ground coriander
Caraway
Fennel seeds
Paprika

CHAPTER 5

THE 28 DAY DETOX DIET PLAN

How to use the plan

This eating plan is designed to give you ideas for daily menus. Use it as the basis for developing your own eating plan, according to your personal tastes and preferences. You do not have to follow it rigidly – you may swap meal plans between different days if you wish. For example, you may want to substitute the lunch from day 14 for the suggested lunch on day 10.

However, the daily menus have been constructed to provide the right balance of protein, carbohydrate, vitamins, minerals and fibre within each day. They incorporate the right mix of foods to ensure you get all the nutrients you need.

For example, you should consume a variety of carbohydrate foods such as quinoa, oats, pulses or fruit within each day, rather than getting all of your carbohydrate from one or two foods. That way, you get a variety of different vitamins, minerals and fibres, which is better for your body.

The key really is variety. Although it may seem easier to stick to the same foods each day, you may miss out on particular nutrients and fail to get maximum benefit from your detox diet. Try to vary your meals as much as possible by following as many of the suggested menus and recipes as you can. You can even make up your own recipes as long as you keep to the principles of the detox diet outlined in Chapter 3.

You will see that suggestions are given for fresh fruit, salad ingredients, seeds and nuts in the daily menu plans. This is really to help give you ideas for varieties you may not otherwise have chosen, as well as ensuring you get a good mixture of nutrients. However, you may substitute other varieties according to season, price and your personal tastes if you wish.

The menus do not specify quantities – and that's for very good reasons. Firstly, everyone has different requirements for calories and nutrients so a blanket recommendation would not suit everyone. In fact, it would probably only suit a very small minority of people! Secondly, this is not a weight-loss diet. The idea is that you eat according to your own needs and to your appetite. Certainly, you should never go hungry or feel that you are depriving yourself of food. Remember that you are restoring your body to full health and that weight loss should be considered as more of a welcome side effect. Eat as much fresh fruit, vegetables, salad and pulses as you wish. These are your real 'fillers'. However, eat sensible amounts of the more calorific foods such as nuts, seeds, grains and oils. Eat them for their nutritional value rather than for their filling power!

Drinks

Aim to drink 6–8 glasses of water each day – that's about 1.5–2 litres – and more during hot weather or on days when you exercise. (See Chapter 3: Simple Principles of the Detox Diet.)

Snacks

Allow yourself a snack whenever you feel hungry. A couple of snacks per day is about right but you can freely eat fresh fruit and vegetables between meals. Here are some ideas for suitable snacks to eat between meals.

- Oatcakes or rice cakes with hummus or tahini.
- Rye crispbreads with a little Manuka honey or nut butter.
- Any type of fresh fruit (bananas in moderation, say every other day).
- Crudités: florets of broccoli and cauliflower, pepper, cucumber, carrot and celery sticks, cherry tomatoes, mangetout, baby sweetcorn, radishes, spring onions.
- A few dried dates, apricots, mango pieces, apple rings or figs (unsweetened and unsulphured varieties).
- A small handful of sultanas or raisins.
- An avocado, halved, stoned and mashed in its skin.
- A small handful of nuts*: almonds, walnuts, peanuts, cashews, pistachios, brazils, pecans.
- A small handful of seeds*: pumpkinseeds, sunflower seeds, sesame seeds.
- A few olives.

* To vary nuts and seeds, toast lightly under a grill for a few minutes to enhance flavour or soak them for an hour and bring out the live enzymes for maximum nutrition and easier digestion.

DAY 1

BREAKFAST

Carrot and apple kick-start (see recipe on page 139)
Mixed seeds, e.g. pumpkinseeds, sunflower seeds, flaxseeds on millet and
oat porridge
Herbal tea

LUNCH

Crudités: cauliflower florets, mangetout, cucumber sticks, celery sticks,
radishes, grapes
Hummus (see recipe on page 71)
Fresh fruit, e.g. strawberries, blueberries, kiwi fruit

EVENING MEAL

Quinoa pilaf with chickpeas and almonds (see recipe on page 123)

DETOX TIP

'I took my own food to work to avoid temptation at the local sandwich bar
– fresh fruit, soup in a flask, rye crispbreads and small packets of nuts were
my mainstay.'

DAY 2

BREAKFAST

Oat porridge with rice, sesame or almond milk (see recipe on page 64)
Raisins, dates or prunes

LUNCH

Vegetable soup (see recipe on page 79)
Rye bread with tahini or nut butter

EVENING MEAL

Spiced rice with pumpkinseeds (see recipe on page 122)
Melon with strawberries and mint (see recipe on page 130)

DETOX TIP

'Like me, you may feel more tired than usual during the first few days, but
that doesn't last long.'

DAY 3

BREAKFAST

Bowl of fresh fruit, e.g. oranges, pineapple and mango
Mixed toasted seeds, e.g. pumpkinseeds, sesame seeds, sunflower seeds

LUNCH

Avocado and walnut salad (see recipe on page 88)
Oranges, satsumas or clementines

EVENING MEAL

Red kidney bean hotpot (see recipe on page 110)
Mixed salad leaves with walnut dressing (see recipe on page 99)

DETOX TIP

'I would make a large bowl of fresh fruit salad in the morning then keep it in the fridge ready for snacking during the rest of the day.'

DAY 4

BREAKFAST

Fresh fruit medley (apple, melon, grapes, kiwi)
Grilled tomatoes and sesame seeds on non-wheat bread toast

LUNCH

Hot pasta with vegetables (see recipe on page 116)

EVENING MEAL

Rice with grilled vegetables (see recipe on page 120)
Mixed nuts and seeds, e.g. walnuts, brazils, pumpkinseeds, sesame seeds
Fresh fruit, e.g. peaches, raspberries, apples

DETOX TIP

'I found that I needed to urinate more often in the first few days. That's a good sign as the body is shedding excess fluid and detoxifying.'

DAY 5

BREAKFAST

Strawberry and raspberry smoothie (see recipe on page 140)
Rye crispbreads with a little honey or nut butter

LUNCH

Jacket potato drizzled with olive oil or essential oil blend
Large mixed salad with pumpkinseeds and toasted almonds
Fresh fruit, e.g. pears, oranges

EVENING MEAL

Vegetable kebabs (use any combination of courgettes, aubergines,
mushrooms, peppers, cherry tomatoes, small onions and broccoli spears)
brushed with olive oil
Cooked quinoa with cashew nuts

DETOX TIP

'I got headaches during the first week, which were a result of cutting down
on caffeine. But they didn't last beyond a few days.'

DAY 6

BREAKFAST

Millet porridge with rice, sesame or almond milk and honey (see recipe on
page 65)

LUNCH

Oatcakes topped with nut butter
Alfalfa sprouts and salad leaves
Fresh fruit, e.g. peaches, apricots, watermelon

EVENING MEAL

Pepper and cashew pilaf (see recipe on page 121)
Strawberry and raspberry smoothie (see recipe on page 140)

DETOX TIP

'Be adventurous and try new ingredients, like millet and quinoa. I asked my
health food store assistant for some tips on what to do with different grains
and pulses.'

DAY 7

BREAKFAST

Freshly squeezed fruit juice
Fresh fruit muesli (see recipe on page 63)

LUNCH

Brown rice and sweetcorn salad (see recipe on page 93)

EVENING MEAL

Red lentil dhal with sunflower seeds (see recipe on page 108)
Fresh fruit, e.g. kiwi fruit and oranges

DETOX TIP

'I began to sleep much better and feel more energetic during the second week!'

DAY 8

BREAKFAST

Apricot and prune compote (soak dried apricots and prunes overnight then stew in a little water)
Add chopped nuts (e.g. brazils, almonds) to serve

LUNCH

Avocado boat (see recipe on page 69)
Slice of non-wheat bread with tahini or nut butter
Orange, satsuma or clementine

EVENING MEAL

Quick supper salad with pumpkinseed dressing (see recipe on page 94)
Fresh fruit, e.g. papaya, mango, peaches

DETOX TIP

'I managed to follow the detox diet on a tight budget. Although I was buying more fruit (which is expensive), I was saving money by not buying booze, chocolate bars and all those convenience foods.'

DAY 9

BREAKFAST

Slice of rye bread with honey
Fresh fruit, e.g. melon, papaya, blueberries

LUNCH

Crudités: broccoli florets, carrot, cucumber or celery sticks, radishes
Rye crispbreads
Olives
Guacamole dip (see recipe on page 72)

EVENING MEAL

Flageolet bean and courgette provençale (see recipe on page 113)
Non-wheat pasta

DETOX TIP

'If you miss bread, choose rye bread or a wheat-free bread. They are much more filling anyway.'

DAY 10

BREAKFAST

Oat porridge with rice, sesame or almond milk (see recipe on page 64)
Chopped dates, figs or prunes

LUNCH

Pineapple rice (see recipe on page 125)
Mixed salad leaves with walnut dressing (see recipe on page 99)
Fresh fruit, e.g. apple, kiwi fruit, mango

EVENING MEAL

Grilled pepper salad (see recipe on page 89)
Steamed quinoa

DETOX TIP

'By day 10 my clothes were feeling looser, which was good, but you must resist the temptation to weigh yourself!'

DAY 11

BREAKFAST

Citrus reviver (see recipe on page 138)
Mixed nuts and seeds, e.g. walnuts, brazils, pumpkinseeds, sesame seeds

LUNCH

Rice and millet salad (see recipe on page 95)
Fresh fruit, e.g. apple, banana, kiwi fruit

EVENING MEAL

Falafel (chickpea 'cakes'; available from most supermarkets)
Large green salad with sliced peaches, avocado, pine nuts and a little
essential oil dressing (see page 97)

DETOX TIP

'Whenever I had a craving for something sweet, I had a piece of fresh fruit,
some dried apricots, or some sesame snaps for a treat. Try also the recipe
for marzipan balls on page 75.'

DAY 12

BREAKFAST

Millet porridge with rice, almond or sesame milk and honey (see recipe on
page 65)
Fresh berries, e.g. raspberries, strawberries, blackberries

LUNCH

Carrot and coriander soup (see recipe on page 78)
Rye bread with tahini or nut butter
Apple or pear

EVENING MEAL

Vegetable and lentil curry (see recipe on page 112)
Brown rice

DETOX TIP

'I threw out the sauce bottles. Instead I enjoyed flavouring my food with
different spices and herbs. Adjust the amounts of spices to suit your own
taste, though.'

DAY 13

BREAKFAST
Freshly squeezed fruit juice
Toasted non-wheat bread with honey

LUNCH
Stir-fried vegetables of your choice with toasted nuts or seeds
Fresh fruit, e.g. papaya, oranges

EVENING MEAL
Non-wheat pasta with lentil bolognese (see recipe on page 117)
Strawberries and rhubarb poached in orange juice

DETOX TIP

'I made good use of my wok – it's a great way of cooking vegetables quickly and keeping in those vitamins. But don't add soy sauce as it's very salty and some brands contain additives.'

DAY 14

BREAKFAST
Bowl of fresh fruit, e.g. papaya, kiwi fruit, grapefruit
Mixed nuts, e.g. almonds, cashews, pecans

LUNCH
Quinoa and rice pilaf (see recipe on page 124)
Mixed salad leaves

EVENING MEAL
Bubble and squeak (see recipe on page 105)
Cool summer fruit salad (see recipe on page 133)

DETOX TIP

'I was really spurred on by how much better my clothes fitted me. In fact, I'd dropped a whole dress size by the end of the 28 day diet.'

DAY 15

BREAKFAST

Mango smoothie (see recipe on page 141)

LUNCH

Rice cakes topped with sliced avocado, tomatoes and rocket
Crudités, e.g. cauliflower and broccoli florets, carrot, cucumber or celery sticks, radishes
Mixed nuts (e.g. pistachios, almonds, brazils, hazelnuts) and seeds (e.g. pumpkinseeds, sunflower seeds)

EVENING MEAL

Tofu and pineapple stir-fry (see recipe on page 127)
Brown rice
Fresh fruit, e.g. mango, papaya, pineapple

DETOX TIP

'Try dandelion tea – it's a great detoxifier. It tastes a bit unusual to start with but you soon get used it.'

DAY 16

BREAKFAST

Muesli with dried fruit (see recipe on page 62)

LUNCH

Green bean and spinach salad (see recipe on page 96)
Non-wheat bread with tahini or nut butter
Melon and sultanas

EVENING MEAL

Cauliflower and potato curry (see recipe on page 106)
Mixed green salad with watercress, baby spinach and rocket and a little garlic and herb dressing (see recipe on page 98)

DETOX TIP

'I kept a large bottle of water on my desk and aimed to have a glass of water every hour.'

DAY 17

BREAKFAST

Millet porridge with rice, almond or sesame milk and honey (see recipe on page 65)

LUNCH

Minestrone soup (see recipe on page 80)
Fresh fruit, e.g. clementines, satsumas, grapes

EVENING MEAL

Quinoa pilaf with chickpeas and almonds (see recipe on page 123)
Cool summer fruit salad (see recipe on page 133)

DETOX TIP

'I found that my skin really started to glow and I looked so well! That's a great incentive to keep going, isn't it?'

DAY 18

BREAKFAST

Sliced pears and apples with sultanas and toasted almonds

LUNCH

Avocado and tomato dip (see recipe on page 70)
Crudités: broccoli florets, carrot, cucumber or celery sticks, radishes
Oatcakes or rice cakes

EVENING MEAL

Citrus salad with pumpkinseeds (see recipe on page 91)
Steamed new potatoes with fresh mint
Melon

DETOX TIP

'Don't buy those bags of ready-prepared salads – the cut vegetables will have lost most of their vitamins. I would buy whole leaves, such as baby spinach, watercress and lamb's lettuce, which are delicious and much better for you.'

DAY 19

BREAKFAST
Fresh fruit muesli with kiwi fruit (see recipe on page 63)

LUNCH
Mixed beans (e.g. red kidney beans, chickpeas, haricot beans, flageolet beans) with raisins, cashew nuts and essential oil dressing (see recipe on page 97)

EVENING MEAL
Stuffed courgettes (see recipe on page 104)
Cooked millet
Baked bananas (see recipe on page 135)

DETOX TIP
'I made a large batch of muesli, kept it in a large jar, then simply added various fruits to it in the morning.'

DAY 20

BREAKFAST
Oat porridge with rice, sesame or almond milk (see recipe on page 64)
Berries, e.g. strawberries, raspberries, blueberries, blackberries

LUNCH
Lentil and vegetable soup (see recipe on page 83)
Mixed nuts, e.g. cashews, almonds, pecans

EVENING MEAL
Guacamole (see recipe on page 72)
Large mixed green salad with a little walnut dressing (see recipe on page 99)
Cooked quinoa

DETOX TIP
'I allowed myself a small glass of white wine at weekends, just to keep my spirits up!'

DAY 21

BREAKFAST
Spiced fruit compote (see recipe on page 134)

LUNCH
Baked potato drizzled with a little olive or pumpkinseed oil
Beansprout and carrot salad: beansprouts, grated carrot, cherry tomatoes,
orange segments and mixed leaves tossed with a little cider vinegar dressing
(see recipe on page 100)

EVENING MEAL
Broccoli and red pepper stir-fry with cashew nuts (see recipe on page 126)
Brown rice
Orange and kiwi fruit salad (see recipe on page 131)

DETOX TIP

'By this stage in the 28 day diet, my insomnia went away! I felt much more
relaxed and was able to sleep without any help.'

DAY 22

BREAKFAST
Slice of rye bread with honey
Oranges or clementines

LUNCH
Mixed leaf salad with avocado (see recipe on page 90)
Fresh fruit, e.g. peaches, nectarines, melon

EVENING MEAL
Mixed bean chilli (see recipe on page 111)
Cooked millet

DETOX TIP

'When I didn't have time to prepare dishes, I simply steamed some
vegetables, added a handful of toasted nuts and drizzled over a little flaxseed
oil. Hey presto!'

DAY 23

BREAKFAST

Freshly squeezed fruit juice
Fresh fruit muesli with grated apple (see recipe on page 63)

LUNCH

Spiced rice with pumpkinseeds (see recipe on page 122)
Fresh fruit, e.g. plums, apricots or nectarines

EVENING MEAL

Pumpkin and sweet potato soup (see recipe on page 85)
Fresh fruit, e.g. peaches, strawberries, pears

DETOX TIP

'I treated myself to a meal out once a fortnight – that satisfied my desire for "normal" food and helped keep my motivation up.'

DAY 24

BREAKFAST

Millet porridge with rice, sesame or almond milk and honey
(see recipe on page 65)

LUNCH

Roasted winter vegetables (see recipe on page 102) with toasted pumpkinseeds
Cooked quinoa

EVENING MEAL

Chickpea, coriander and lime salad (see recipe on page 92)
Baked bananas (see recipe on page 135)

DETOX TIP

'I actually stopped using ordinary salt altogether by the end of the 28 day detox. Instead, I flavoured my food with lemon juice, lime juice and herb salt.'

DAY 25

BREAKFAST
Carrot and apple kick-start (see recipe on page 139)
Rye crispbread with nut butter or tahini

LUNCH
Steamed millet
Ratatouille made with onions, garlic, aubergines, courgettes, tomatoes, peppers and fresh basil
Mixed seeds, e.g. pumpkinseeds, sunflower seeds, sesame seeds

EVENING MEAL
Asparagus and lemon soup (see recipe on page 81)
Non-wheat pasta with olives, tossed in a little olive oil

DETOX TIP
'Instead of spreading butter or margarine on my bread and crispbreads, I used a little hummus or nut butter, which tasted delicious.'

DAY 26

BREAKFAST
Bowl of fresh fruit, e.g. nectarines, mango, apricots
Mixed seeds (e.g. pumpkinseeds, sunflower seeds) or nuts (e.g. almonds, hazelnuts)

LUNCH
Pasta and cannellini soup (see recipe on page 84)
Mango, papaya or pineapple

EVENING MEAL
Roasted Mediterranean vegetables (see recipe on page 103)
Cooked quinoa

DETOX TIP
'For a really quick meal, I would simply toss peppers, courgettes, onions and mushrooms (whatever I had to hand really) in a little olive oil, sprinkle with herbs or garlic, then bake in a hot oven until just tender.'

DAY 27

BREAKFAST
Muesli with dried fruit (see recipe on page 62)
Freshly squeezed fruit juice

LUNCH
Crudités: broccoli florets, carrot, cucumber or celery sticks, radishes
Red pepper and almond dip (see recipe on page 74)
Bowl of fresh fruit, e.g. nectarines, apricots, melon

EVENING MEAL
Millet pilaf with almonds (see recipe on page 128)

DETOX TIP
'One of the biggest changes I made was getting into the habit of having breakfast. At first it felt wrong but after only a week, I found that I had a lot more energy in the mornings. I also felt less hungry in the evenings and automatically ate less for supper.'

DAY 28

BREAKFAST
Oat porridge with rice, sesame or almond milk and chopped dates
(see recipe on page 64)

LUNCH
Non-wheat pasta with tomato and vegetable sauce (see recipe on page 118)
Mango smoothie (see recipe on page 141)

EVENING MEAL
Butter bean and tomato casserole (see recipe on page 109)
Steamed new potatoes with fresh mint drizzled with a little flaxseed oil

DETOX TIP
'At first, I was worried about feeling hungry on the diet. But the foods I ate were so filling and satisfying that I can honestly say I never felt deprived.'

CHAPTER 6
THE RECIPES

Recipe notes

- The recipes make enough for 4 servings so they may be used as the basis for family meals. Increase or decrease the quantities if you wish to serve more or fewer people. Remember, though, you can always save any remaining portions in the fridge or freezer.

- Keep salt to a minimum. Season only where necessary and, preferably, at the end of cooking. Use sea salt, a low-sodium salt or a herb seasoning salt.

- Where olive oil is specified in the recipes, use extra-virgin olive oil.

- For all other seed and nut oils, use a cold-pressed (ideally organic) variety.

- Essential oil blends contain a mixture of cold-pressed seed oils rich in omega-3 and omega-6 fatty acids.

- Although not essential, try to use organic ingredients wherever possible (see Chapter 3: Simple Principles of the Detox Diet, page 21).

- Don't use seed and nut oils for frying as very high temperatures produce potentially harmful changes in the oils. Instead, add at the end of cooking (e.g. blended into soups) or drizzle on salads, bread, pasta or potatoes. Sauté vegetables in a little stock or water.

- Nuts and seeds benefit enormously from a light toasting under the grill (or a few minutes in a hot oven) to bring out their full nutty flavour.

- Where stock is stated in the recipes, either use homemade (see recipe on page 86) or a ready-made fresh vegetable stock. Avoid stock cubes as most brands contain too much salt.

- Use a non-wheat pasta, such as rice millet pasta or corn pasta. Follow the cooking instructions on the packet. In most cases, the cooking time is slightly shorter compared with wheat pasta.

BREAKFASTS

Muesli with dried fruit

Makes 4 servings

175–200 g (6–7 oz) porridge oats (use millet flakes if you are sensitive to gluten)

2 tablespoons (30 ml) oat bran

60 g (2 oz) raisins

60 g (2 oz) dates, chopped

60 g (2 oz) dried apricots, chopped

60 g (2 oz) flaxseeds, ground

1. Put all the ingredients in a bowl and mix well.

2. Serve with rice, sesame or almond milk.

3. You can make larger quantities and store in an airtight container.

Fresh fruit muesli

Makes 4 servings

175–200 g (6–7 oz) cereal flakes

e.g. porridge oats, rye millet and rice flakes

2 tablespoons (30 ml) oat bran

2 tablespoons (30 ml) seeds, e.g. sunflower, pumpkin, ground flaxseeds

2 tablespoons (30 ml) flaked almonds or hazelnuts

450 g (1 lb) fresh fruit, e.g. strawberries, coarsely

grated apple or pear, sliced kiwi

1. Place the cereal flakes in serving bowls and cover with 200–250 ml (7–8 fl oz) water. Leave to soak overnight.

2. Add the oat bran and seeds and top with the fresh fruit.

3. Serve with soya, rice, oat or almond milk.

Oat porridge

Makes 4 servings

175 g (6 oz) porridge oats

250 ml (9 fl oz) rice, sesame or almond milk

250 ml (9 fl oz) water

4 teaspoons (20 ml) Manuka honey or maple syrup

Optional: handful of raisins, sultanas or chopped dates

1. Mix the oats, milk and water in a saucepan. Bring to the boil and simmer for approximately 5 minutes, stirring continuously.

2. Serve with the honey or maple syrup and raisins or dates if you wish.

Millet porridge

Makes 4 servings

175 g (6 oz) millet flakes

225 ml (9 fl oz) rice, sesame or almond milk

225 ml (9 fl oz) water

Vanilla essence or nutmeg to taste

4 teaspoons (20 ml) Manuka honey or maple syrup

1. Mix the oats, milk, water and vanilla or nutmeg in a saucepan.

2. Bring to the boil and simmer for 4 or 5 minutes, stirring continuously.

3. Serve with the honey or maple syrup.

SNACKS

Crudités

Crudités make excellent snacks. Accompany them with one of the dips on the following pages and you have a quick, healthy meal. Use only the freshest vegetables. Almost any vegetables that can be eaten raw are suitable. Here are some suggestions.

Florets of broccoli
Florets of cauliflower
Strips of red, yellow, orange or green pepper
Carrot sticks
Celery sticks
Small mushrooms
Cherry tomatoes
Crisp chicory leaves
Mangetout
Baby sweetcorn
Radishes
Spring onions
Cucumber, cut into strips
Courgette, cut into strips

Avocado boat

Makes 1 serving

½ avocado

1 tomato, finely chopped

A few toasted pumpkinseeds

Freshly ground black pepper

A few leaves of fresh basil, torn

1. Remove the avocado stone. Roughly mash the avocado flesh in its skin.

2. Add the chopped tomato and pumpkinseeds; season with black pepper to taste.

3. Scatter over the torn basil leaves.

Avocado and tomato dip

Makes 1 serving

½ red onion, finely chopped

1 clove of garlic, crushed

Pinch of ground cumin

1–2 teaspoons (5–10 ml) olive oil

1 tomato, chopped

½ avocado, chopped

Freshly ground black pepper

1. Place the red onion, garlic, cumin and olive oil in a shallow pan set over a low heat. Warm for about 5 minutes to allow the flavours to infuse and the onion to soften.

2. Add the chopped tomato and avocado.

3. Season with the black pepper.

Hummus

Makes about 600 ml (1 pint)

225 g (8 oz) chickpeas, soaked overnight

(or 2 x 400 g tins, drained and rinsed)

2 garlic cloves

2 tablespoons (30 ml) olive oil

4 tablespoons (60 ml) tahini

Juice of 1.5 lemons

Pinch paprika

Freshly ground black pepper

1. Drain then cook the chickpeas in plenty of water for about 60–90 minutes or according to directions on the packet. Drain, reserving the liquid.

2. Purée the cooked chickpeas with the remaining ingredients with enough of the cooking liquid to make a creamy consistency.

3. Taste and add more black pepper or lemon juice if necessary.

4. Chill in the fridge.

Guacamole (Avocado Dip)

Makes about 600 ml (1 pint)

2 ripe avocados

2 tablespoons (30 ml) lemon or lime juice

1 small onion, finely chopped

1 clove of garlic, crushed

2 tomatoes, chopped

A few coriander or parsley sprigs, finely chopped

Freshly ground black pepper

1. Mash the avocado flesh with the lemon or lime juice.

2. Add the remaining ingredients, mixing well.

3. Check the seasoning, adding a little more black pepper or lemon juice if necessary. Chill.

Aubergine dip

Makes about 600 ml (1 pint)

1 aubergine

2 tablespoons (30 ml) lemon juice

2 tablespoons (30 ml) olive oil

2 tablespoons (30 ml) chopped parsley

1 tablespoon (15 ml) tahini

1 clove of garlic, crushed

Freshly ground black pepper

1. Pre-heat the oven to 200° C/ 400° F/Gas mark 6.

2. Prick the aubergine all over with a fork, put on a baking tray and bake for about 40 minutes until soft. Alternatively, prick then cook in a microwave on full power for approximately 3 minutes.

3. Allow to cool then purée in a blender or food processor with the remaining ingredients. Chill.

Red pepper and almond dip

Makes about 600 ml (1 pint)

2 red peppers

3 cloves of garlic, crushed

60 g (2 oz) ground almonds

2 tablespoons (30 ml) olive oil

Freshly ground black pepper

1. Steam the peppers for about 15–20 minutes until tender. Drain and remove the stems and seeds.

2. Purée the cooked peppers with the remaining ingredients. Chill.

Marzipan balls

This is a healthy treat for those moments when you fancy something sweet.

Makes 20 small balls

80 g (3 oz) almonds

2 tablespoons (30 ml) Manuka honey

1–2 teaspoons water

Ground cinnamon

1. Grind the almonds finely and knead with the honey and water to a smooth mass.

2. Form small balls and roll them in the ground cinnamon.

SOUPS

Carrot and Coriander soup

Makes 4 servings

1 onion, chopped

1 clove of garlic, chopped

675 g (1.5 lbs) carrots, sliced

900 ml (1.5 pints) vegetable stock

Salt and freshly ground black pepper

1–2 tablespoons fresh coriander, chopped

1 tablespoon (15 ml) olive oil

1. Place the onion, garlic and carrots in a large saucepan. Add the stock and bring to the boil, then reduce the heat and simmer for 15 minutes until the carrots are tender.

2. Season with the salt, freshly ground black pepper and add the fresh coriander and olive oil.

3. Liquidise in a blender or food processor.

Vegetable soup

Makes 4 servings

1 onion, chopped

1 garlic clove, crushed

1 litre (1.8 pints) vegetable stock

750 g (1.5 lbs) vegetables of your choice (see below)

1 tablespoon (15 ml) olive oil

Season with salt and freshly ground black pepper

1 tablespoon (15 ml) fresh mixed herbs, e.g. chives, parsley, marjoram, or 1 teaspoon (5 ml) dried herbs

Vegetables: chopped potato, sliced courgettes, sliced carrots, diced pumpkin, chopped green beans, frozen peas, broccoli florets, cauliflower florets

1. Place the onion, garlic, olive oil, vegetable stock and vegetables in a large saucepan. Bring to the boil and simmer for about 20 minutes or until the vegetables are soft.

2. Turn off the heat. Add the olive oil, seasoning and herbs.

3. For a smooth soup, liquidise in a blender or food processor or hand blender. For a chunky, thick soup, liquidise half the soup and return to the pan.

Minestrone soup

Makes 4 servings

1 onion, chopped

2 garlic cloves, crushed

1 litre (1.8 pints) vegetable stock

2 carrots, chopped

125 g (4 oz) courgettes, peas, green beans

2 teaspoons dried basil

1 tin (400 g) haricot beans

125 g (4 oz) small pasta shapes

600 ml (1 pint) passata (smooth sieved tomatoes) or tinned chopped tomatoes

1 tablespoon (15 ml) olive oil

1. Sauté the onions and garlic in the olive oil for 5 minutes.

2. Add the vegetables, herbs and remaining stock and simmer for about 10 minutes. Add the beans, pasta and passata and continue cooking for a further 10 minutes.

3. Turn off the heat. Stir in the olive oil.

Asparagus and lemon soup

Makes 4 servings

2 onions, finely chopped

450 g (1 lb) asparagus, trimmed and sliced

300 g (10 oz) potato, peeled and sliced

1 litre (1.8 pints) water

Salt and freshly ground black pepper

1 tablespoon (15 ml) chopped fresh oregano

Juice of 1 lemon

1. Place the onions, asparagus, potato and water in a large saucepan.

2. Bring to the boil and simmer for 10 minutes until the vegetables are tender.

3. Add the black pepper, oregano and lemon juice and simmer for 2 minutes. Blend in a liquidiser or food processor.

4. Serve warm or chilled.

Broccoli and bean soup

This sounds like an unusual combination but it works really well. The mild flavoured flageolet beans and potato give the soup a creamy texture. Broccoli is one of the most nutritious vegetables, full of vitamin C, iron, folic acid and cancer-fighting phytochemicals.

Makes 4 servings

4 spring onions, sliced

1 garlic clove, crushed

2 teaspoons (10 ml) mild curry powder

1.5 litres (2.5 pints) vegetable stock

1 medium potato, chopped

450 g (1 lb) broccoli florets

400 g (14 oz) can flageolet beans, drained

1. Place the onions, garlic and curry powder in a saucepan with about 150 ml (0.25 pint) of the stock. Bring to the boil and simmer for about 5 minutes.

2. Add the remaining stock, the potato and broccoli and simmer for 15–20 minutes.

3. Add the beans then purée the soup in a blender or food processor (in small batches if necessary).

Lentil and vegetable soup

Makes 4 servings

225 g (8 oz) red lentils

1.5 litres (2.5 pints) vegetable stock

2 carrots, sliced

1 onion, chopped

2 potatoes, diced

450 g (1 lb) chopped vegetables of your choice, e.g. swede, turnip, parsnip, courgette, cauliflower florets, leek

Salt and freshly ground black pepper

1. Place the lentils in a large saucepan with the vegetable stock and boil for 10 minutes. Alternatively, cook in a pressure cooker for 3 minutes then release the steam.

2. Add the vegetables, bring back to the boil and simmer for a further 15–20 minutes until the vegetables and lentils are soft (or cook in the pressure cooker for a further 3 minutes).

3. Season with salt and pepper.

Pasta and cannellini soup

Makes 4 servings

1 large onion, chopped

2 celery stalks, sliced

1 teaspoon paprika

400 g (14 oz) can chopped tomatoes

1 litre (1.75 pints) vegetable stock

2 carrots, diced

125 g (4 oz) wheat-free pasta

1 tin (420 g) cannellini or haricot beans, drained

1 tablespoon (15 ml) olive oil

Salt and freshly ground black pepper

1. Place the onion, celery, paprika, tomatoes, vegetable stock and carrots in a large saucepan. Bring to the boil and simmer for 10 minutes until the vegetables are soft.

2. Add the pasta and beans and cook for a further 7–10 minutes.

3. Stir in the olive oil. Season to taste with salt and freshly ground black pepper.

Pumpkin and sweet potato soup

Makes 4 servings

1 onion, chopped

1 clove of garlic, chopped

675 g (1.5 lbs) pumpkin flesh, cubed

450 g (1 lb) sweet potatoes, peeled and cubed

1 teaspoon (5 ml) fresh ginger, grated

2 teaspoons (10 ml) ground coriander

1.5 litres (2.5 pints) vegetable stock

1 tablespoon (15 ml) olive oil

Freshly ground black pepper

1. Put the onion, garlic, pumpkin, sweet potato, ginger and ground coriander in a large saucepan.

2. Add the stock and bring to the boil, then reduce the heat and simmer for 25–30 minutes until the vegetables are tender.

3. Add the olive oil. Season with salt and freshly ground black pepper and liquidise in a blender or food processor.

Vegetable stock

Use this stock for making soups, stews and casseroles and in any recipes that call for stock. It has a better flavour than stock made with stock cubes and is much lower in salt. Make double quantities and freeze the remainder.

Makes 600 ml (1 pint)

900 ml (1.5 pints) water

2 onions, sliced

2 carrots, roughly sliced

2 celery sticks, halved

1 leek, halved

2 bay leaves

2 sprigs of thyme

2 sprigs of parsley

8 black peppercorns

Pinch of sea salt to season

1. Put the water, vegetables, herbs and seasonings in a large saucepan.

2. Bring to the boil and simmer gently for at least 1 hour.

3. Leave to cool and then strain.

SALADS

Salads are extremely simple to make, need no cooking, and are bursting with vitamins, minerals, and antioxidant nutrients. Adjust the quantities of the ingredients according to what you have available and to your own preferences.

Avocado and walnut salad

Makes 4 servings

2 avocados, peeled, stoned and halved

1 tablespoon (15 ml) lemon juice

2–3 handfuls of salad leaves, e.g. rocket, watercress, lettuce

125 g (4 oz) walnut halves

FOR THE DRESSING:

1 tablespoon (15 ml) walnut oil

1 tablespoon (15 ml) olive oil

2 teaspoons (10 ml) cider vinegar

1 teaspoon (5 ml) lemon juice

1. Cut the avocados into slices and turn gently in the lemon juice to stop them discolouring.

2. Place the mixed salad leaves in the serving dish.

3. Arrange the avocado slices on top and sprinkle over the walnuts.

4. Shake the dressing ingredients together in a screw-topped jar. Drizzle over the salad.

Grilled pepper salad

Makes 4 servings

1 red pepper

1 yellow pepper

1 green pepper

1 orange pepper

Olive oil for brushing

1 tablespoon (15 ml) fresh basil leaves, roughly torn

2 tablespoons (60 g) black olives

2 tablespoons (30 ml) olive oil

1 tablespoon (15 ml) cider vinegar

175 g (6 oz) mixed salad leaves

1. Cut the peppers into quarters and remove the seeds. Place on a grill tray and brush lightly with olive oil. Grill, skin-side up, until just beginning to char.

2. Cut into strips and place in a bowl.

3. Add the basil leaves and black olives.

4. In a separate bowl or screw-top jar, mix the olive oil and vinegar together.

5. Toss the peppers in the dressing. Arrange on a bed of salad leaves.

Mixed leaf salad with avocado

Makes 4 servings

225 g (8 oz) mixed salad leaves, e.g. oak leaf lettuce, baby spinach, rocket, endive

Handful of fresh mint, finely chopped (optional)

2 courgettes, finely sliced

2 avocados, peeled, stoned and sliced

1 tablespoon (15 ml) olive oil

1 tablespoon (15 ml) essential oil blend

1 teaspoon (5 ml) cider vinegar

1 teaspoon (5 ml) lemon juice

1. Combine the salad leaves, mint and courgettes in a large bowl.

2. Arrange the sliced avocado on top.

3. In a separate jar or bowl combine the oils, vinegar and lemon juice. Spoon over the salad. Serve immediately.

Citrus salad with pumpkinseeds

Makes 4 servings

125 g (4 oz) mixed salad leaves

2 oranges, peeled and segmented

1 pink grapefruit, peeled and segmented

6 shallots (or 1 red onion), peeled and finely sliced

2 tablespoons (30 ml) fresh coriander, chopped

60 g (2 oz) pumpkinseeds, toasted

FOR THE DRESSING:

2 tablespoons (30 ml) olive oil

1 tablespoon (15 ml) cider vinegar

½ teaspoon (2.5 ml) wholegrain mustard

1 clove of garlic, crushed

Salt and freshly ground black pepper

1. Place the salad ingredients in a large bowl and toss lightly.

2. Place the dressing ingredients in a screw-top jar and shake well.

3. Pour over the salad, toss well and serve immediately.

Chickpea, coriander and lime salad

Makes 4 servings

500 g (1 lb 2 oz) cooked chickpeas

(or use 2 x 400 g / 14 oz cans chickpeas,

drained and rinsed)

1 red onion, thinly sliced

1 red pepper, finely chopped

2 tablespoons (30 ml) fresh coriander, chopped

2 garlic cloves, crushed

3 tablespoons (45 ml) olive oil

Juice of 1 lime

1. Drain and rinse the canned chickpeas.

2. Combine with the sliced onion, chopped pepper and chopped coriander.

3. In a screw-top jar, mix together the crushed garlic, olive oil and lime juice.

4. Pour over the chickpea salad, mix well and chill in the fridge. This is best prepared at least 2 hours in advance before eating so the chickpeas have time to absorb the flavours.

Brown rice and sweetcorn salad

Makes 4 servings

350 g (12 oz) rice

4 spring onions, chopped

2 red peppers, chopped

125 g (4 oz) sultanas

60 g (2 oz) flaked toasted almonds

225 g (8 oz) sweetcorn

1. Cook the rice according to directions on the packet. Drain if necessary, rinse in cold water and drain again.

2. Place in a large bowl and combine with the remaining ingredients.

Quick supper salad with pumpkinseed dressing

Makes 4 servings

250 g cooked pinto beans, or any other variety

(or use a 400 g/14 oz can)

125 g (4 oz) bean sprouts

2 large tomatoes, chopped

2 sticks celery, sliced

2 tablespoons (30 ml) chopped fresh parsley

1 tablespoon (15 ml) pumpkinseed oil

1 tablespoon (15 ml) olive oil

1 tablespoon (15 ml) cider vinegar

2 tablespoons (30 ml) sunflower seeds

1. Drain and rinse the beans. Combine with the chopped vegetables and parsley.

2. Mix the pumpkinseed oil, olive oil and vinegar together and drizzle over the salad.

3. Scatter over the sunflower seeds.

Rice and Millet Salad

Makes 4 servings

60 g (2 oz) brown rice, cooked

60 g (2 oz) millet, cooked

1 red pepper, finely diced

1 yellow pepper, finely diced

2 celery sticks, finely diced

4 spring onions, finely diced

2 tomatoes, skinned and finely chopped

60 g (2 oz) walnuts or cashew nuts, chopped

2 tablespoons (30 ml) olive oil

1 garlic clove, crushed

1 tablespoon (15 ml) lemon juice

3 tablespoons (45 ml) parsley, chopped

2 tablespoons (30 ml) mint, chopped

Freshly ground black pepper

1. Combine the cooked grains in a bowl and mix in the peppers, celery, spring onions, tomatoes and walnuts or cashews.

2. In a separate bowl, mix the olive oil, garlic, lemon juice, parsley and mint. Season to taste with the freshly ground black pepper.

3. Add the dressing to the salad and mix well. This salad is best chilled in the fridge before serving.

Green bean and spinach salad

Makes 4 servings

225 g (8 oz) thin green beans, cut into 5 cm (2 inch) lengths

500 g (1 lb 2 oz) cooked mixed beans of your choice *

(or use 2 x 400 g/14 oz cans mixed beans)

2 tablespoons (30 ml) olive oil

2 tablespoons (30 ml) cider vinegar

125 g (4 oz) baby spinach leaves

* You may use any combination of haricot, butter, pinto, cannellini, red kidney beans or chickpeas.

1. Boil or steam the thin green beans until just tender – about 4 minutes. Refresh in cold water and drain.

2. Mix together the green beans, cooked mixed beans, olive oil and vinegar in a bowl.

3. Place the spinach leaves in the bottom of the serving bowl and pile the bean mixture on top.

Dress up a salad

A dressing transforms a salad or plate of vegetables into something special and is a great way to get those essential oils in your diet. Here are some

Essential oil dressing

2 tablespoons (30 ml) seed oil blend

1 tablespoon (15 ml) olive oil

1 tablespoon (15 ml) cider vinegar or lemon juice

Freshly ground black pepper, to taste

1. Shake the ingredients together in a screw-top jar.

2. Serving suggestion: as a dressing for leaf and bean salads, with avocado or with steamed vegetables.

Garlic and herb dressing

60 ml (2 fl oz) cider vinegar

2 tablespoons (30 ml) orange juice

1 tablespoon (15 ml) olive oil

1 garlic clove, crushed

1 tablespoon (15 ml) chopped fresh parsley

1 tablespoon (15 ml) chopped fresh tarragon

1. Place the ingredients in a screw-top jar and shake well to combine.

2. Serving suggestion: as a dressing for lettuce and other leaf salads; on coleslaw; with avocado; with steamed green vegetables such as broccoli and green beans.

Walnut dressing

1 tablespoon (15 ml) cold-pressed sunflower oil

1 teaspoon (5 ml) walnut oil

Juice of ½ lemon

1 tablespoon (15 ml) walnuts, toasted and finely chopped

Season with freshly ground black pepper

1. Place the ingredients in a screw-top jar and shake well to combine.

2. Serving suggestion: as a dressing for lettuce and other leaf salads.

Cider vinegar dressing

1 tablespoon (15 ml) cider vinegar

3 tablespoons (45 ml) olive oil

1 tablespoon (15 ml) chopped fresh oregano

or 1 teaspoon (5 ml) dried oregano

Pinch of salt and freshly ground black pepper, to taste

1. Place the ingredients in a screw-top jar and shake well to combine.

2. Serving suggestion: as a dressing for leafy salads; tomatoes; raw or roasted peppers; with steamed asparagus; on cold pasta salads.

VEGETABLE MAIN DISHES

Roasted winter vegetables

You can use any seasonal vegetables of your choice.

Makes 4 servings

450 g (1 lb) pumpkin, peeled and thickly sliced

2 carrots, peeled and halved

4 parsnips, peeled and cut into quarters

1 large sweet potato, peeled and sliced

1 small swede, peeled and cut into wedges

A few sprigs of rosemary

2 garlic cloves, crushed

Salt and freshly ground black pepper

2 tablespoons (30 ml) olive oil

1. Prepare the vegetables and place in a large roasting tin.

2. Place the herbs between the vegetables and sprinkle with the crushed garlic and pepper. Drizzle over the oil and turn the vegetables gently so they are coated in a little oil.

3. Roast in a pre-heated oven at 200° C/ 400° F/Gas mark 6 for 30–40 minutes until the vegetables are tender.

Roasted Mediterranean vegetables

You can use any seasonal vegetables of your choice.

Makes 4 servings

2 courgettes, thickly sliced

8 shallots

1 aubergine, sliced

1 red pepper, cut into strips

1 yellow pepper, cut into strips

125 g (4 oz) cherry tomatoes

A few sprigs of rosemary or oregano

2 garlic cloves, crushed

Salt and freshly ground black pepper

2 tablespoons (30 ml) olive oil

1. Prepare the vegetables and place in a large roasting tin.

2. Place the herbs between the vegetables and sprinkle with the crushed garlic and pepper. Drizzle over the oil and turn the vegetables gently so they are coated in a little oil.

3. Roast in a pre-heated oven at 200° C/ 400° F/Gas mark 6 for 30–40 minutes until the vegetables are tender.

Stuffed courgettes

Makes 4 servings

4 courgettes

1 red onion, finely chopped

½ teaspoon (2.5 ml) cumin seeds

Pinch of paprika

12–15 cherry tomatoes

4 carrots or parsnips, grated

1. Pre-heat the oven to 190° C/ 375° F/ Gas mark 5.

2. Cut the courgettes in half lengthways. Using a teaspoon remove the flesh leaving 6 mm (0.25 inch) in the shell.

3. Put the chopped onion in a little water with the cumin seeds to soften for a few minutes and to bring out the flavour of the cumin. Add the paprika and tomatoes. Cook for a further 2–3 minutes.

4. Add the grated carrot and courgette flesh and cook for a further 5 minutes until softened.

5. Pile the mixture into the courgette shells. Place on foil in an ovenproof dish. Bake until the courgette shells are soft, approximately 30–45 minutes.

Bubble and squeak

Makes 4 servings

450 g (1 lb) potatoes

450 g (1 lb) green leafy vegetables, e.g. any combination

of cabbage, spinach, Brussels sprouts, spring greens

3–4 tablespoons (45–60 ml) rice/ almond milk

Season with salt, freshly ground black pepper,

chopped parsley

1. Peel and chop the potatoes. Steam for 15–20 minutes until tender. Drain.

2. Meanwhile, prepare the green vegetables. Steam for 10 minutes until soft. Drain, reserving liquid for soups, stock, etc.

3. Mash the potatoes and vegetables with the milk and seasoning.

4. Spoon into a small ovenproof dish, level the surface and grill until the top is crispy.

Cauliflower and potato curry

Makes 4 servings

2 tablespoons (30 ml) water or vegetable stock

2 onions, chopped

450 g (1 lb) cauliflower, broken into florets

1 tablespoon (15 ml) curry powder

8 new potatoes, cut into halves

1 tablespoon (15 ml) tomato purée

60 ml (2 fl oz) water

175 g (6 oz) frozen peas

1. Heat the water or stock in a large pan and cook the onions for 5 minutes until soft.

2. Add the cauliflower, curry powder and potatoes. Cook for 1 minute.

3. Add the tomato purée, water and peas and cook until the vegetables are tender and the curry has thickened.

PULSE DISHES

Red lentil dhal with sunflower seeds

Makes 4 servings

2 onions, chopped

2 tablespoons (30 ml) water or vegetable stock

3–4 garlic cloves, crushed

1 teaspoon ground cumin

2 teaspoons ground coriander

1 teaspoon turmeric

350 g (12 oz) red lentils

1.2 litres (2 pints) water

125 g (4 oz) sunflower seeds

2 tablespoons (30 ml) oil

Salt to season

Handful of fresh coriander or parsley, finely chopped

1. Sauté the onion in the water or stock for a few minutes. Add the garlic and spices and cook for a further minute.

2. Add the lentils and water and bring to the boil. Cover and simmer for about 20 minutes. Alternatively, cook in a pressure cooker for 3 minutes then turn off the heat.

3. Stir in the sunflower seeds, olive oil, salt and fresh coriander or parsley.

Butter beans and tomato casserole

This nutritious one-pot meal is simplicity itself. Use any other vegetables at hand (e.g. onions, mushrooms) in place of the leeks if you prefer.

Makes 4 servings

1 tablespoon (15 ml) water or vegetable stock

2 leeks, sliced

1 tin (400 g/14 oz) chopped tomatoes

2 x 400 g (2 x 14 oz) cans butter beans, drained

150 ml (0.25 pint) vegetable stock

1. Sauté the leeks in the water for about 5 minutes until they are almost soft.

2. Add the remaining ingredients, stir and bring to the boil. Simmer for a further 10–15 minutes or until the casserole has thickened.

3. Accompany with new potatoes.

Red kidney bean hotpot

Makes 4 servings

2 tablespoons (30 ml) water

1 onion, chopped

1 garlic clove, chopped

1 red pepper, chopped

125 g (4 oz) mushrooms, sliced

400 g (14 oz) can tomatoes

2 x 400 g (2 x 14 oz) cans red kidney beans,

rinsed and drained

1 teaspoon mixed herbs

250 ml (8 fl oz) vegetable stock

2 teaspoons (10 ml) cornflour

1. Dry-fry the onion, garlic and red pepper in the water over a high heat for 3–4 minutes.

2. Add the mushrooms, tomatoes (roughly broken up), beans, herbs and vegetable stock. Stir well and bring to the boil.

3. Blend the cornflour with a little water to make a smooth paste then stir into the hotpot to thicken the sauce. Simmer for 10 minutes.

Mixed bean chilli

Makes 4 servings

1 large onion, chopped

2 or 3 garlic cloves, crushed

2 tablespoons (30 ml) water or vegetable stock

Pinch of chilli powder, according to your taste

1 tablespoon each of tomato purée and paprika

400 g (14 oz) can chopped tomatoes

400 g (14 oz) can red kidney beans, drained

400 g (14 oz) can cannellini beans, drained

500 g (1 lb) mixed sliced vegetables

(e.g. carrots, peppers, courgettes, etc.)

1. Sauté the onion, garlic and chilli for 5 minutes in the water or vegetable stock.

2. Add the tomato purée and paprika and cook for 2 minutes.

3. Add the tinned tomatoes, beans and vegetables. Stir and bring to the boil. Simmer for 20 minutes until the vegetables are tender.

Vegetable and lentil curry

Lentils add protein, fibre and iron to the curry. Vary the vegetables according to what you have available.

Makes 4 servings

2 tablespoons (30 ml) water or vegetable stock

1 large onion, sliced

1 teaspoon (5 ml) each of cumin, coriander,

turmeric and chilli powder

(Alternatively use 1 tablespoon curry powder)

2 garlic cloves, crushed

225 g (8 oz) red lentils

750 ml (1.25 pints) water

900 g (2 lbs) vegetables (e.g. cauliflower, courgettes, mushrooms, okra, carrots, tomatoes)

1. Sauté the onion in the water or stock for 5 minutes.

2. Add the spices and the garlic and continue cooking for 2 minutes.

3. Add the red lentils and water. Cover and simmer for 10 minutes. Add the vegetables and continue cooking for 20 minutes or until the vegetables are just tender.

Flageolet bean and courgette provençale

Makes 4 servings

1 tablespoon (15 ml) olive oil

2 onions, sliced

2 garlic cloves, crushed

450 g (1 lb) courgettes, sliced

2 x 400 g (2 x 14 oz) cans flageolet beans, drained

400 g (14 oz) can tomatoes

1 teaspoon (5 ml) dried oregano

150 ml (5 fl oz) vegetable stock

1. Heat the oil in a large pan and sauté the onion for about 5 minutes until softened.

2. Add the garlic and courgettes and cook for a further 5 minutes.

3. Add the remaining ingredients. Cover and simmer for another 10 minutes.

PASTA DISHES

Hot pasta with vegetables

This basic pasta recipe takes less than 15 minutes to prepare. You simply add whatever fresh or frozen vegetables you have handy to the pasta pot and – hey presto! Ideal for quick nutritious suppers and attractive enough to serve to guests at dinner. Any leftovers are also good served cold as a salad.

Makes 4 servings

350 g (12 oz) non-wheat pasta

2 tablespoons (30 ml) olive oil, blended seed oil or pesto sauce

450 g (1 lb) chopped vegetables of your choice*

* Choose any of these vegetables: strips of red, green or yellow peppers, broccoli florets, sliced mushrooms, peas, sliced courgettes.

1. Cook the pasta in plenty of boiling water according to the directions on the packet. If you prefer cooked vegetables, add them during the last 5 minutes of cooking (otherwise add them raw in step 3). Drain.

2. While hot, combine the pasta with the olive oil or pesto and raw vegetables if you prefer.

Pasta with lentil bolognese

Makes 4 servings

350 g (12 oz) non-wheat pasta

3 tablespoons (45 ml) water or vegetable stock

1 onion, chopped

2 carrots, finely chopped

1 large courgette, finely chopped

400 g (14 oz) can chopped tomatoes

400 g (14 oz) can brown or green lentils

1 teaspoon (5 ml) mixed herbs

1. Cook the pasta in plenty of boiling water according to the directions on the packet.

2. Sauté the vegetables in the water or stock for about 5 minutes until softened. Add the tomatoes, lentils and herbs. Cook for a further 5–10 minutes until the sauce thickens slightly.

3. Drain the pasta and place on the serving dish. Top with the lentil bolognese.

Pasta with tomato and vegetable sauce

Makes 4 servings

350 g (12 oz) non-wheat pasta

3 tablespoons (45 ml) water or vegetable stock

1 onion, chopped

2 garlic cloves, crushed

2 or more vegetables from the list below*

400 g (14 oz) can chopped tomatoes

2 tablespoons (30 ml) tomato purée

1 tablespoon (15 ml) chopped fresh or 1 teaspoon (5 ml) dried basil

1. Cook the pasta in plenty of boiling water according to the directions on the packet.

2. Meanwhile, heat the water or stock in a large frying pan. Add the onion, garlic and prepared vegetables and cook for about 5 minutes until softened. Add the chopped tomatoes, tomato purée and basil. Cook for 5 minutes or until the vegetables are tender but still firm.

* Suitable vegetables for the sauce: 225 g (8 oz) asparagus, chopped into 4 cm lengths; 2 courgettes, sliced; 1 red, green or yellow pepper, chopped; 225 g (8 oz) broccoli florets; 150 g (5 oz) mangetout; 1 small aubergine, finely chopped; 125 g (4 oz) mushrooms, sliced; 125 g (4 oz) peas; 125 g (4 oz) French beans, chopped into 4 cm lengths.

DISHES WITH GRAINS

Rice with grilled vegetables

Makes 4 servings

300 g (10 oz) brown rice

3 peppers (red, yellow, green), deseeded

and cut into quarters

2 medium red onions, sliced

225 g (8 oz) mushrooms

2 small courgettes, cut in half lengthways

Olive oil, for brushing

2 tablespoons (30 ml) fresh thyme, chopped

For the dressing:

3 tablespoons (45 ml) olive oil

2 tablespoons (30 ml) lemon juice

2 cloves of garlic, crushed

Freshly ground black pepper

1. Put the rice in a pan of boiling water. Water level should be about 2.5 cm (1 inch) above the rice. Stir, lower the heat and simmer for 20–30 minutes until tender.

2. To make the dressing mix together the olive oil, fresh lemon juice, garlic and black pepper. Set aside while grilling vegetables.

3. Arrange vegetables on a grill rack. Brush with olive oil and grill for 8–10 minutes until tender and slightly brown. Turn occasionally and brush again.

4. Drain the rice mix in half the dressing. Spoon into a serving dish, arrange the vegetables on top, then pour over the remaining dressing. Scatter over the chopped thyme.

Pepper and cashew pilaf

Makes 4 servings

2 tablespoons (30 ml) water or vegetable stock

1 onion, chopped

2 garlic cloves, crushed

4 celery sticks, chopped

1 red, yellow and green pepper, sliced

300 g (10 oz) brown rice

900 ml (1.5 pints) vegetable stock

125 g (4 oz) cashew nuts, broken

Handful of fresh parsley, chopped

Salt and freshly ground pepper to taste

1. Heat the water or stock in a large pan and sauté the onion, garlic, celery and peppers for 5 minutes.

2. Add the brown rice and stir for another 2–3 minutes.

3. Add the vegetable stock, bring to the boil then simmer for 20–25 minutes until the liquid has been absorbed and the rice is cooked.

4. Stir in the cashews and parsley, then season to taste with the salt and freshly ground black pepper.

Spiced rice with pumpkinseeds

Makes 4 servings

½ teaspoon (2.5 ml) cumin seeds

1 teaspoon (5 ml) ground coriander

300 g (10 oz) brown rice

900 ml (1.5 pints) vegetable stock

225 g (8 oz) frozen peas

4 tablespoons (60 ml) pumpkinseeds, lightly toasted

1. Dry-fry the cumin seeds, ground coriander and brown rice in a large saucepan for about 2 minutes.

2. Add the vegetable stock, bring to the boil and simmer for 20–25 minutes or until the rice is tender and the liquid has been absorbed.

3. Add the peas and cook for a further 3 minutes. Stir in the pumpkinseeds and heat through before serving.

Quinoa pilaf with chickpeas and almonds

Makes 4 servings

2 tablespoons (30 ml) water or vegetable stock

1 onion, chopped

1 stick cinnamon

4 cardamom pods

2 cloves of garlic, crushed

1 red pepper, chopped

2 courgettes, sliced

225 g (8 oz) quinoa

600 ml (1 pint) vegetable stock or water

250 g (9 oz) cooked chickpeas

(or use a 400 g/14 oz can of chickpeas, drained and rinsed)

60 g (2 oz) toasted flaked almonds

60 g (2 oz) pumpkinseeds

Handful of fresh coriander or parsley, chopped

1. Heat the water in a large saucepan and sauté the onion with the cinnamon stick and cardamom pods for 2 minutes.

2. Add the garlic, peppers and courgettes and cook for a further 2 minutes. Add the quinoa, vegetable stock and cooked chickpeas. Stir and bring to the boil. Reduce the heat and simmer for about 20 minutes until the liquid has been absorbed and the quinoa is cooked.

3. Pile the pilaf on to the serving plates. Scatter over the almonds and pumpkinseeds. Sprinkle with chopped coriander or parsley.

Quinoa and rice pilaf

Makes 4 servings

1 tablespoon (15 ml) olive oil

1 onion, chopped

125 g (4 oz) brown rice

125 g (4 oz) quinoa

600 ml (1 pint) vegetable stock

150 g (5 oz) peas

Salt and freshly ground black pepper

Handful of fresh parsley, chopped

Squeeze of lemon juice

1. Place the oil in a large saucepan and add the onion. Allow to infuse for 5 minutes.

2. Add the rice, quinoa and stock and stir well. Bring to the boil, reduce the heat then simmer for about 20–25 minutes until the liquid has been absorbed and the grains are tender.

3. Add the peas and cook for a further 3 minutes. Season with salt and pepper. Stir in the parsley and lemon juice. Fluff with a fork.

Pineapple rice

Makes 4 servings

300 g (10 oz) brown rice

900 ml (1.5 pints) vegetable stock

1 onion, chopped

½ teaspoon (2.5 ml) turmeric

225 g (8 oz) fresh pineapple

(or use 225 g/8 oz can chopped pineapple in juice, drained)

60 g (2 oz) currants

1. Place the rice, stock, onion and turmeric in a large saucepan.

2. Bring to the boil and simmer for 20–25 minutes until the rice is tender and the liquid has been absorbed.

3. Add the pineapple and currants. Heat through before serving.

Broccoli and red pepper stir-fry with cashew nuts

Makes 4 servings

2 tablespoons (30 ml) water

1 garlic clove, crushed

2.5 cm (1 inch) root ginger, peeled and finely grated

4 spring onions, chopped

2 red peppers, sliced

450 g (1 lb) broccoli florets

125 g (4 oz) button mushrooms

125 g (4 oz) cashew nuts

1 tablespoon (15 ml) sesame oil

1. Heat the water in a wok. Add the garlic, ginger and spring onions and stir-fry for 2 minutes.

2. Add the other vegetables to the wok. Stir-fry for 3–4 minutes.

3. Add the cashew nuts, drizzle over the sesame oil and heat through.

Tofu and pineapple stir-fry

Makes 4 servings

2 tablespoons (30 ml) water

2 garlic cloves, crushed

2.5 cm (1 inch) piece fresh ginger, chopped

1 red pepper, chopped

4 spring onions, chopped

225 g (8 oz) mushrooms, sliced

125 g (4 oz) bean sprouts

200 g (7 oz) can pineapple pieces, drained

4 tablespoons (60 ml) water

1 teaspoon (5 ml) cornflour

350 g (12 oz) firm tofu, cubed

1. Heat the water in a wok and stir-fry the garlic and ginger for 1 minute.

2. Add the red pepper, onions, mushrooms, bean sprouts and pineapple, and stir-fry for 2 minutes.

3. Blend the water with the cornflour and pour over the vegetables and stir quickly until the sauce has thickened. Transfer on to a serving dish.

4. Stir-fry the tofu in the wok for 1 minute, turning frequently, and arrange on the vegetables.

Millet pilaf with almonds

Makes 4 servings

2 tablespoons (30 ml) water

1 large onion, chopped

2 carrots, diced

2 teaspoons (10 ml) ground coriander

1 garlic clove, crushed

175 g (6 oz) millet

600 ml (1 pint) vegetable stock

225 g (8 oz) broccoli florets

60 g (2 oz) sultanas

Freshly ground black pepper to taste

60 g (2 oz) toasted flaked almonds

1. Heat the water in a saucepan and cook the onion for 5 minutes.

2. Add the carrots, ground coriander and garlic and cook for a further 5 minutes. Add the millet and vegetable stock, bring to the boil, cover and simmer for 15–20 minutes until the water has been absorbed.

3. Add the broccoli and cook for 5 minutes. Stir in the raisins and season with freshly ground black pepper.

4. Serve scattered with the toasted flaked almonds.

FRUIT DESSERTS

Melon with strawberries and mint

Makes 4 servings

225 g (8 oz) strawberries

4 sprigs of mint

16 blanched almonds

2 small Ogen or galia melons

1. Cut the strawberries into halves or quarters and place in a bowl. Roughly tear the mint leaves and add to the strawberries.

2. Add the almonds.

3. Cut the melons in half. Scoop out the seeds and fill the cavities with the strawberries.

Orange and kiwi fruit salad

Makes 4 servings

4 oranges

4 kiwi fruit

1–2 teaspoons (5–10 ml) orange flower water

Manuka honey to taste

1. Carefully remove the peel and pith from the oranges then cut into segments. Put in a bowl.

2. Peel the kiwi fruit and slice thinly. Add to the bowl.

3. Add the orange flower water and honey to taste and mix gently.

Winter fruit salad

Makes 4 servings

125 g (4 oz) dried fruit mixture, e.g. apricots, peaches, apples, figs

250 ml (8 fl oz) freshly squeezed orange juice

1 ruby grapefruit, segmented

1 orange, segmented

1 pear, chopped

1. Place dried fruit and orange juice in a large bowl and leave in the fridge overnight.

2. Add the remaining fruit. Serve.

Cool summer fruit salad

Makes 4 servings

125 g (4 oz) strawberries

125 g (4 oz) grapes

4 kiwi fruit, sliced

4 apricots, chopped

150 ml (5 fl oz) freshly squeezed fruit juice

1. Combine the prepared fruit and fruit juice in a bowl.

2. Spoon into individual bowls.

Spiced fruit compote

Makes 4 servings

250 g (8 oz) mixed dried fruits, e.g. apples, apricots, prunes, peaches, cranberries

1 stick of cinnamon

3 cardamom pods, lightly crushed

300 ml (10 fl oz) freshly squeezed orange or apple juice

300 ml (10 fl oz) hot water

1. Place the fruit in a bowl with the cinnamon stick and cardamom pods.

2. Pour over the juice and water. Leave to cool then place in the fridge overnight.

3. Remove the spices before serving.

Baked Bananas

Makes 4 servings

4 large bananas

4 tablespoons (60 ml) water

2 tablespoons (30 ml) Manuka honey or maple syrup

1/2 teaspoon mixed spice

60 g (2 oz) raisins

1 tablespoon (15 ml) lemon juice

1. Slice the bananas into 2.5 cm (1 inch) chunks.

2. Place in a baking dish and combine with the remaining ingredients.

3. Bake at 200° C/ 400° F/Gas mark 6 for 15 minutes.

JUICES AND SMOOTHIES

Citrus reviver

Citrus juice is a superb liver and intestinal cleanser. It's also particularly good for relieving fluid retention and digestive problems. Rich in vitamin C and antioxidant bioflavanoids, this drink is also an excellent antiseptic that will help to ward off colds, coughs and sore throats.

Makes 2 drinks

1 grapefruit

4 oranges

2 lemons

2 limes

1. Peel the fruit then blend the ingredients together.

2. Drink immediately.

Ginger booster

Ginger is a gentle cleanser and is good for beating off colds and flu. It also relieves digestive problems and nausea. The beta-carotene in the carrots is a cancer-fighting antioxidant that will also benefit your skin.

Makes 2 drinks

4 carrots

2 teaspoons (10 ml) chopped fresh ginger

2 oranges, peeled

1. Juice all the ingredients and drink immediately.

Carrot and apple kick-start

This is a great detoxifying juice, excellent for the skin and useful for lowering blood pressure. The powerful diuretic effects of carrots and celery help relieve fluid retention.

Makes 2 drinks

6 carrots

4 apples, cut in quarters

4 sticks of celery

1. Blend all the ingredients together and drink immediately.

Strawberry and raspberry smoothie

Bursting with vitamin C, this is a wonderful pick-me-up when summer berries are in season.

Makes 2 drinks

300 ml (0.5 pint) freshly squeezed orange juice

1 banana

125 g (4 oz) strawberries

125 g (4 oz) raspberries

1. Place all the ingredients in a blender and blend until smooth.

Mango smoothie

Mangoes are rich in cancer-fighting beta-carotene and are terrific immune system boosters. One drink provides more than your daily requirement of beta-carotene.

Makes 2 drinks

400 g (14 oz) or 2 medium sized mangoes

1 banana

300 ml (0.5 pint) almond milk

1. Blend all the ingredients together and drink immediately.

BAKING

There's even room on the detox diet for a little sweet indulgence. Here are some recipes for delicious bakes that are wheat-free and dairy-free. Please note that they contain honey (and fruit) instead of sugar, and one recipe contains eggs. These ingredients do not support the elimination of toxins, so it would be a good idea to limit how often you indulge in these tasty but healthy treats. If during the 28 days you are finding the detox unbearable, then an occasional treat of your choice will not totally ruin the plan.

Fruitcake

Perfect for the festive season (or any celebration), this cake is made without sugar, dairy fat, eggs and wheat. Instead, it contains highly nutritious ingredients such as fresh apples, almonds, honey and dried fruit, which provide natural sweetness and moisture. It also has an intriguing tangy flavour and a less cloying texture than traditional fruitcake. Enjoy!

Makes 12 slices

125 ml (4 fl oz) sunflower oil

4 tablespoons (60 ml) honey

2 apples, peeled and grated

125 g (4 oz) ground almonds

Grated zest and juice of 2 oranges

Grated zest and juice of 1 lemon

250 g (9 oz) wheat-free flour*

2 teaspoons (10 ml) baking powder (preferably wheat-free)

125 g (4 oz) raisins

125 g (4 oz) sultanas

*Available from most supermarkets. Most brands contain rice flour and potato starch.

1. Pre-heat the oven to 170º C/ 325º F/Gas mark 4.

2. Mix together the sunflower oil and honey.

3. Add the grated apples, almonds and the orange and lemon rind and juice and mix well.

4. Fold in the flour, baking powder, raisins and sultanas.

5. Oil and line with parchment a 20 cm (8 inch) round cake tin. Spoon in the cake mixture. Bake for 50–60 minutes.

6. Check that the cake is done by inserting a skewer or knife into its centre. It should come out clean. Allow the cake to cool slightly in the tin, then turn out onto a wire rack to cool completely.

Almond shortbread

Honey is a wonderful substitute for sugar in this recipe so the end result is slightly less crumbly than – but equally as delicious as – traditional shortbread. The ground almonds not only add essential oils and protein but also give this shortbread a wonderfully moist texture.

Makes 12 slices

125 g (4 oz) dairy-free spread

125 g (4 oz) honey

150 g (5 oz) rice flour or ground rice

125 g (4 oz) wheat-free flour

125 g (4 oz) ground almonds

1. Pre-heat the oven to 160° C/ 325° F/Gas mark 3. Line a baking tray with baking parchment and brush with oil.

2. Cream the dairy-free spread and honey in a bowl or food processor until smooth.

3. Stir the flours onto the creamed mixture, add the ground almonds and combine using a wooden spoon or process until the mixture comes together into a soft ball.

4. Gather the dough together with your hands, then transfer the mixture onto the baking tray, pressing it down to a thickness of about 1 cm (0.5 inches) in a neat square shape, approximately 20 cm x 20 cm (8 inches x 8 inches).

5. Bake for about 15–20 minutes until very pale golden. Be careful not to over-bake otherwise the shortbread may be a little dry.

6. Remove from the oven then leave to cool on the baking sheet for 10 minutes. Cut into about 12 slices, then transfer them to a wire rack to cool completely.

Date, apple and walnut cake

This cake is sweetened with dates and sultanas, which provide extra fibre and potassium. It includes eggs but as this cake is eaten only occasionally, it will not ruin your detox efforts.

Makes 12 slices

125 g (4 oz) dairy-free spread

200 g (7 oz) dates

2 eating apples, peeled and grated

Pinch of freshly grated nutmeg

½ teaspoon (2.5 ml) ground cinnamon

2 eggs

250 g (9 oz) wheat-free flour

2 teaspoons (10 ml) baking powder (preferably wheat-free)

175 ml (6 fl oz) soya, rice, sesame or almond milk

125 g (4 oz) sultanas

85 g (3 oz) walnuts, chopped

1. Pre-heat the oven to 180° C/ 350° F/Gas mark 4. Line and lightly oil a round 20 cm (8 inch) cake tin.

2. Cover the dates with boiling water, leave to soak for 10 minutes, drain, then roughly mash with a fork to a lumpy pulp.

3. In a mixing bowl or food processor, blend the dairy-free spread, dates, apples and spices. Add the eggs and mix or process until combined. Fold in the flour, baking powder, alternating with the milk. Finally fold in the sultanas and walnuts. The mixture will be quite soft.

4. Transfer the mixture into the prepared tin. Bake for 35 minutes or until golden and firm to the touch.

5. Remove from the oven and leave to cool in the tin for 15 minutes before turning on to a wire rack. to cool completely.

Cranberry muffins

This cake is sweetened with dates and sultanas, which provide extra fibre and potassium. It includes eggs but as this cake is eaten only occasionally, it will not ruin your detox efforts.

Makes 12 muffins

175 g (6 oz) wheat-free flour

125 g (4 oz) cornmeal

1 tablespoon (15 ml) baking powder (preferably wheat-free)

2 tablespoons (30 ml) honey

2 tablespoons (30 ml) sunflower oil

175 ml (6 fl oz) soya, almond, rice or sesame milk

150 ml (5 fl oz) apple juice

225 g (8 oz) fresh cranberries (or 85 g (3 oz) dried cranberries)

1. Pre-heat the oven to 200° C/ 400° F/Gas mark 6.

2. Sift the flour, cornmeal and baking powder into a bowl. Mix together the honey, oil, milk and apple juice in a large jug. Pour into the bowl and mix all the ingredients together to make a fairly runny batter. Add the cranberries and combine together.

3. Spoon the mixture into 12 non-stick bun tins or paper cases.

4. Bake in the oven for 15 minutes or until golden. Leave to cool for 5 minutes, then transfer to a wire rack.

ENTERTAINING

Eating with friends should be equally enjoyable on the detox diet. The following recipes are not only healthy, in keeping with the detox principles, but are tasty and attractive enough to impress the most sceptical guest.

Roasted vegetable tart with sunflower seeds

This tart makes a great centrepiece and works equally well with other seasonal vegetables. For summer entertaining, try courgettes, aubergines and plum tomatoes instead of the root vegetables. If you don't like making pastry, you can buy a wheat-free pastry mix from supermarkets or health food stores.

Makes 4 servings

Oat Pastry:

225 g (8 oz) porridge oats

60 g (2 oz) ground almonds

25 g (1 oz) chopped toasted hazelnuts

or sesame seeds

1 teaspoon (5 ml) dried mixed herbs

150 g (5 oz) dairy-free spread

FILLING:

2 red onions, cut into chunks

1 red pepper, cut into 2.5 cm (1 inch) squares

½ butternut squash, peeled, deseeded and

chopped into 2.5 cm (1 inch) cubes

175 g (6 oz) sweet potato, peeled and

chopped into 2.5 cm (1 inch) cubes

2 carrots, peeled and cut into

2.5 cm (1 inch) pieces

2 tablespoons (30 ml) olive oil

1 clove of garlic, crushed

A few sprigs of rosemary

Freshly ground black pepper

200 g (7 oz) tofu

1 tablespoon (15 ml) cider vinegar

150 ml (0.25 pints) soya, rice, sesame or

almond milk

2 tablespoons (30 ml) sunflower seeds

1. Pre-heat the oven to 200° C/ 400° F/ Gas mark 6.

2. Process the oats in a food processor until fine, then add the almonds, hazelnuts or sesame seeds, dried herbs and dairy-free spread. Process until the mixture is well combined.

3. Press the pastry over the base and sides of an oiled 20 cm (8 inch) flan tin. Bake in the oven for 10 minutes.

4. Put all of the vegetables in a roasting tin together with the garlic, rosemary and black pepper. Drizzle over the oil, toss well and roast in the oven for about 30 minutes until tender.

5. Put the tofu, vinegar and milk into a blender or food processor and blend until smooth.

6. Put the roast vegetables in the flan case then spoon over the tofu mixture. Sprinkle the sunflower seeds over the top and bake for 20–25 minutes.

Little aubergine rolls filled with tomatoes and courgettes

These aubergine rolls are very easy to make and will certainly impress your guests. You can vary the filling by adding other chopped vegetables, such as mushrooms and red peppers, and by substituting other varieties of nuts for the walnuts.

Makes 4 servings

1 large aubergine

2 tablespoons (30 ml) olive oil

Freshly ground black pepper

3 large tomatoes

1 onion, finely chopped

1 clove garlic, crushed

1 courgette, diced

40 g (1.5 oz) chopped walnuts

1 tablespoon (15 ml) basil leaves, torn

1 tablespoon (15 ml) sun-dried tomato paste

8 black olives, chopped

1. Pre-heat the oven to 180° C/ 350° F/Gas mark 4.

2. Using a sharp knife, cut the aubergines lengthways into 8 thin slices, about 5 cm (0.25 inches) thick. Lay the aubergine slices on a lightly oiled baking tray. Lightly brush with olive oil and season with the freshly ground black pepper.

3. Cook in the oven for 15 minutes.

4. Remove the skin from the tomatoes,* deseed if you have time, then cut into dice.

5. Heat 1 tablespoon olive oil in a pan and sauté the onion and garlic for 5 minutes. Add the diced tomatoes and courgettes, walnuts, torn basil leaves and tomato paste and cook for 5 minutes. Add the chopped olives.

6. Place an equal amount of filling on each aubergine slice. Roll each aubergine slice into a cylinder. Place in a lightly oiled baking dish and brush with a little olive oil. Cover the dish with foil and bake for 20 minutes.

*The easiest way to remove the skin from tomatoes is to cut a small cross in the bottom of them. Place in a small bowl and cover with boiling water. Leave for 30 seconds then plunge into a bowl of cold water. You should then be able to pull the skin off with the tip of a knife.

Grilled cashew nut and sun-dried tomato cakes with red peppers and fennel

These nutty 'mini-burgers' make a great starter as well as a main course. You can use other types of nuts, such as ground almonds or walnuts, if you wish, and, for children, serve them in a wholemeal bun.

Makes 4 servings

175 g (6 oz) brown rice

1 onion, finely chopped

1 tablespoon (15 ml) olive oil

1 clove garlic, crushed

200 g (7 oz) cashew nuts, lightly toasted

1 tablespoon (15 ml) dried basil

1 tablespoon (15 ml) sun-dried tomato paste

Sea salt and freshly ground black pepper

6 tablespoons (90 ml) porridge oats

1 large head of fennel, trimmed and thinly sliced

2 large red peppers, deseeded and cut into large pieces

A few sprigs of fresh parsley

1. Put the rice into a saucepan with 400 ml (14 fl oz) water. Bring to the boil, turn down the heat and simmer for 40 minutes until the rice is tender and the water has been absorbed.

2. Cook the onion in the oil for 5 minutes, then add the garlic and cook for a further 2 minutes.

3. Put the cooked rice in a food processor with the onions, garlic, cashew nuts, basil, tomato paste and sea salt and pepper to taste. Process until the mixture just holds together. The mixture should be fairly firm.

4. Divide into 8 and form each portion into a patty. Place the oats in a small bowl and dip each patty into the oats, coating all over.

5. Place the patties on a baking tray lined with foil and brush both sides with olive oil. Add the sliced red pepper and fennel.

6. Cook for 5–7 minutes under a hot grill until the patties are crisp and golden and the vegetables lightly browned.

7. Arrange the cashew nut patties on 4 serving plates with the grilled vegetables around them. Garnish with sprigs of fresh parsley.

Baked butternut squash with sunflower seeds

This stunning dish is sure to impress even the most sceptical guests. Not only does it look good but it is plentiful in the antioxidants beta-carotene and vitamin C. Serve it with steamed green vegetables, such as green beans or broccoli, or a delicious leafy salad.

Makes 4 servings

1 large butternut squash

3 tablespoons (45 ml) olive oil

125 g (4 oz) rice or quinoa

300 ml (0.5 pint) vegetable stock or water

1 onion, finely chopped

1 red pepper, deseeded and cut into small pieces

2 carrots, peeled and grated

2 tomatoes, skinned and chopped

1 teaspoon (5 ml) dried thyme

3 tablespoons (45 ml) sunflower seeds, lightly toasted

1. Pre-heat the oven to 200° C/ 400° F/ Gas mark 6.

2. Cut the butternut squash in half and place cut side up on an oiled baking tray. Brush with a little of the olive oil and bake for 35 minutes until the flesh is tender.

3. Cook the rice or quinoa in the stock or water until the liquid has been absorbed and the grains are tender. When the squash is cooked, remove the seeds and scoop out most of the flesh.

4. Heat the remaining olive oil in a pan, add the onion, pepper and carrots and sauté over a moderate heat until soft, about 10 minutes. Add the tomatoes, cooked rice or quinoa, thyme and sunflower seeds and mix well.

5. Spoon the mixture into the butternut squash shells and return to the oven for a further 15 minutes.

Honeyed vanilla pears

The delicate flavours of this dessert complement perfectly any of the main meals above. Conference pears work particularly well in this recipe.

Makes 4 servings

4 ripe pears

4 tablespoons (60 ml) clear honey

1 strip lemon peel

1 strip orange peel

Juice of ½ lemon

1 vanilla pod, split lengthways

4 tablespoons (60 ml) blackcurrant coulis (ready bought)

1. Peel the whole pears carefully with a vegetable peeler, making them look as smooth as possible. You can leave the stalks on. Put them in a small saucepan so they fit snugly together.

2. Cover with water. Add the honey, the lemon and orange peel and the lemon juice. Scrape the seeds from the vanilla pod into the pan and add the pod itself.

3. Bring the pan to the boil, reduce the heat, cover and simmer for about 15 minutes (depending on the size of the pears) until just cooked. Allow to cool in the cooking liquor.

4. Remove the pears. Heat the remaining liquor to a rapid boil and reduce until the syrup has thickened.

5. Place the pears on individual serving plates. Spoon a little syrup over each pear and add a swirl of the blackcurrant coulis.

Apple and blackberry crumble

Makes 4 servings

2 large cooking apples, peeled, cored and sliced

125 g (4 oz) blackberries

2 tablespoons (30 ml) water

4 tablespoons (60 ml) clear honey

60 g (2 oz) flaked almonds, crushed

60 g (2 oz) oats

25 g (1 oz) rice flour

60 g (2 oz) dairy-free spread

1. Pre-heat the oven to 190º C/ 375º F/Gas mark 5.

2. Put the prepared apples, blackcurrants and water into an ovenproof dish. Stir in 2 tablespoons (30 ml) of the honey.

3. Place the flaked almonds, oats, rice flour, dairy-free spread and the remaining honey in a bowl and mix together with your fingers until you have a sticky crumb mixture. Alternatively, blend in a food processor for 20 seconds.

4. Spread the oat crumble over the fruit and bake in the oven for about 25 minutes until the topping is golden. Do not over-bake otherwise the topping will become too hard.

CHAPTER 7

DETOX AND BEYOND

Congratulations on completing the 28 day detox! You should now be reaping the rewards and feeling a good deal healthier than you did before. The chances are that you now want to maintain the new, healthier you. Going back to old eating habits would undo all that good work and you would lose many of the benefits you have gained.

So, think of the 28 day detox as a blueprint for your long-term eating plan. Now that you have got the hang of eating healthily, you can easily incorporate the main elements from this 28 day diet into your regular diet. Of course, you need not stick to the detox principles as rigidly as you have been. You can allow a little more room for manoeuvre now that you have rid your body of old toxins. Here is a guide to staying healthy beyond the 28 day detox.

- Keep to the detox diet principles at least 75 per cent of the time.

- Reintroduce certain foods that you have missed to fill the remaining 25 per cent. For example, you may wish to include ordinary wheat bread or a wheat breakfast cereal in your diet. That should be fine provided you continue to listen to your body.

  If you notice any symptoms, such as bloating or sluggishness, then cut back or eliminate.

- It's best to reintroduce foods one at a time rather than eating them all at once. That way, you will be able to work out those which cause you unpleasant symptoms. Keep a food diary if you can, noting down what you eat and how you feel.

- If you suspect a food allergy or intolerance (e.g. to dairy or gluten) you should consult a qualified nutritional practitioner for professional advice.

- Allow yourself those little indulgences – whether it's chocolate, cheese or wine – without feeling guilty. Most people who have completed the 28 day detox find that their craving is satisfied after eating or drinking only a very small amount. It is surprising how your taste buds change after eating super-healthily for 28 days. Where before you may have eaten a whole chocolate bar (or more!) you may well find that a couple of squares of chocolate now do the trick.

- Continue to listen to your body. If a certain food or drink doesn't feel 'right' or simply doesn't appeal, then don't have it. You should now be much more in tune with your body than you were 28 days ago.

- Do not take the cleansing herbal supplements (such as milk thistle and kelp) for longer than 3 months.

Can I follow the diet plan for longer than 28 days?

There are no hard and fast rules as to how long you should follow the detox diet. The exact length of time really depends on your level of toxicity and how you feel. You usually start to see and feel results after one or two weeks – you may find that you sleep better, have more energy or lose excess weight – but it normally takes 28 days to really reap the benefits. You may continue to follow the diet programme for longer than 28 days if you wish, provided you are feeling well and that you include a wide variety of foods from the permitted list (see Chapter 3: Simple Principles of the Detox Diet, page 21). After all, it takes 3 months to fully detox, regenerate new blood cells, body tissues and new skin cells. However, you will achieve most of the benefits after 28 days.

How often can I use the 28 day detox diet plan?

Clearly, this is not a quick-fix diet that you stick to for a while only to lapse back to old ways. The aim is to adapt the principles of the 28 day detox diet to your long-term eating habits.

However, no one's perfect and sometimes it is easy to let good habits slide a little. For example, during stressful periods, on holiday or during the Christmas festivities, you may not eat as healthily as usual. Toxins may begin to accumulate and your system will be overworked again. You will start to recognise those symptoms of toxin build-up.

That's the time to take stock and go back on the 28 day detox diet. You may need to do this once every 6 months or once a year, for example, as part of your new year's resolution. Whenever you feel the time is right for you.

It may not always be necessary to do the full 28 day detox. You may feel that a week or two is enough to restore your energy and health. Or you may even find that all you need to do is to cut back on certain foods or drinks for a while, for example wheat, alcohol or coffee.

The main message is: listen to your body and respond accordingly.

Maintenance

Many of you have asked me if I could give you some recipes for meals you can enjoy after the first 28 days of the detox, when you want to be a little less strict. So here they are. The recipes in this section are what I call 'maintenance' recipes – they are not as strict as those in the 28-day plan, and may include poultry, fish or low-fat dairy products. They are still well balanced but give you a little more room for manoeuvre. Use them for everyday eating or entertaining.

What to eat

As well as all the foods permitted on the strict detox, you can now reintroduce certain foods. These include:

- Low-fat yoghurt and fromage frais
- Skimmed or semi-skimmed milk
- Cottage cheese and other low-fat cheeses
- Wholemeal bread
- Wholegrain breakfast cereals
- Chicken, turkey and lean meat
- White fish and oily fish

Pancakes with fresh fruit

Makes 10–12 pancakes

PANCAKES:

70 g (2 oz) plain white flour

70 g (2 oz) plain wholemeal flour

2 eggs

250 ml (8 fl oz) soya, rice, almond, oat or skimmed milk

A little rapeseed oil or oil spray for frying

FILLING:

Sliced bananas, sliced strawberries, apple puree with raisins, lightly crushed raspberries, frozen berry mixture (thawed), chopped mango, or sliced nectarines or peaches

Natural bio-yoghurt, to serve

1. Place the flours, eggs and milk in a liquidiser and blend to make a smooth batter.

2. Heat a nonstick frying pan over a high heat. Spray with oil spray or add a few drops of oil. Pour in enough batter to coat the pan thinly and cook for 1–2 minutes until golden brown on the underside.

3. Turn the pancake and cook the other side for 30–60 seconds.

4. Turn out on a plate, cover and keep warm while you make the other pancakes.

5. Serve with any of the suggested fresh fruit fillings and bio-yoghurt.

Broccoli soup

Makes 4 servings

450 g (1 lb) broccoli florets

1 onion, chopped

450 ml (¾ pint) vegetable stock

450 ml (¾ pint) skimmed or non-dairy milk

2 teaspoons (10 ml) cornflour, blended with a little water

A little low-sodium salt and freshly ground black pepper to taste

40 g (1½ oz) toasted flaked almonds

1. Place the onion, broccoli and vegetable stock in a saucepan. Bring to the boil and simmer for about 15 minutes until the vegetables are soft. Liquidise the soup using a hand blender or food processor.

2. Return to the saucepan with the milk, and then stir in the cornflour blended with a little water. Bring to the boil, stirring, and then simmer gently for a minute or two.

3. Serve in individual bowls, sprinkling each portion with the toasted almonds.

Thai chicken and coconut

Makes 4 servings

2 chicken breasts cut into strips

Zest and juice of 1 lime

400 ml (14 fl oz) coconut milk

400 ml (14 fl oz) hot chicken or vegetable stock

1 stem of lemon grass, cut into strips

2.5 cm (1 in) fresh ginger, peeled and grated

1 red chilli, finely chopped (optional)

2 tablespoons (30 ml) chopped fresh coriander leaves

1. In a shallow dish, sprinkle the lime juice over the chicken pieces, cover and leave to marinate in the fridge for at least 30 minutes.

2. Place the remaining ingredients in a large saucepan and heat until boiling. Add the chicken pieces and lime juice. Reduce the heat and simmer for 15 minutes.

3. Ladle into 4 bowls and sprinkle over the coriander leaves.

Sweetcorn and butter bean chowder with green chilli cornbread

Makes 4 servings

Chowder:

2 tablespoons (30 ml) extra virgin olive oil

1 onion, chopped

1 clove garlic, crushed

2 potatoes, peeled and diced

600 ml (1 pint) vegetable stock

600 ml (1 pint) skimmed milk

420 g (14 oz) tinned sweetcorn, drained

420 g (14 oz) tinned butter beans, drained

Freshly ground black pepper

1. Preheat the oven to 180°C/350°F/Gas mark 4.

2. First make the cornbread. Mix together the cornmeal, baking powder and salt in a large bowl.

In a separate bowl combine the eggs, oil and soya milk.

3. Add the wet mixture to the corn meal mixture and mix together. Add the chopped chillies and pour into a lightly oiled 20 cm x 20 cm baking dish.

4. Bake for 25 minutes or until the cornbread is coming away from the sides of the dish and it is risen and golden. While the cornbread is baking, make the chowder.

5. Heat the olive oil in a large pan. Add the onion and garlic and cook over a moderate heat for 5 minutes. Add the potatoes and the stock. Bring to the boil, reduce the heat then simmer for 10 minutes. Add the remaining ingredients and simmer for a further 10 minutes, stirring occasionally. Season with freshly ground pepper to taste.

6. Serve piping hot with the cornbread.

Chicken and mushroom salad with spicy sesame dressing

Makes 4 servings

125 g (4 oz) pack ready-washed salad leaves

1 cucumber, sliced diagonally

A small handful of chopped fresh mint

4 skinless boneless chicken breasts

12 shitake mushrooms

DRESSING:

125 ml (4 fl oz) rice vinegar

1 tablespoon (15 ml) Dijon mustard

4 tablespoons (60 ml) rapeseed oil

2 tablespoons (30 ml) sesame oil

2 teaspoons (10 ml) soy sauce

4 spring onions, chopped

1. To make the dressing: Whisk the vinegar and mustard in a bowl. Gradually whisk in both oils, then the soy sauce. Mix in the spring onions.

2. Place the chicken and mushrooms in a large glass baking dish. Pour half the dressing over and turn to coat. Cover and chill for at least 30 minutes.

3. Reheat the grill. Remove chicken and mushrooms from marinade and cook under the grill until cooked through, about 4 minutes per side for the chicken, about 2 minutes per side for the mushrooms. Slice the cooked chicken and halve the mushrooms.

4. Combine the salad leaves, cucumber and mint in large bowl. Pour enough dressing over salad to coat and toss gently. Transfer to large plate and spoon the chicken slices and mushrooms on top.

Greek salad with fennel

Makes 4 servings

1 romaine (cos) lettuce

1 small bulb of fennel

1 cucumber

2 large tomatoes

1 green, red or orange pepper

1 red onion

115 g (4 oz) black kalamata olives

175 g (6 oz) feta cheese

DRESSING:

4 tablespoons (60 ml) extra virgin olive oil

Juice of 1 lemon

A small bunch of flat-leaf parsley, chopped

A little low-sodium salt and freshly ground black pepper, to taste

1. Cut the lettuce into wide ribbons. Halve and thinly slice the fennel, discarding the tough inner 'core'. Cut the cucumber lengthways in half then half again, and then slice thickly. Cut the tomatoes into quarters. Remove the seeds from the pepper and slice it thinly. Slice the onion thinly.

2. Put the prepared vegetables into a large bowl. Add the feta cheese and olives.

3. Whisk the dressing ingredients together in a small bowl. Pour the dressing over the salad and toss well.

Grilled salmon with niçoise salad

Makes 4 servings

3 eggs

125 g (4 oz) fine green beans, trimmed and halved

2 'Little Gem' lettuces

1 red onion, thinly sliced

225 g (8 oz) cherry tomatoes, halved

4 tablespoons (60 ml) black olives

4 x 125 g (4 oz) salmon steaks

1 lemon, sliced into wedges

DRESSING:

3 tablespoons (45 ml) extra virgin olive oil

1 tablespoon (15 ml) lemon juice

½ teaspoon (2.5 ml) Dijon mustard

1 small clove of garlic, crushed

1. Place the eggs in a saucepan of cold water. Bring to the boil and cook for 5 minutes. Drain and plunge into cold water, then peel. Steam or boil the green beans for 2 minutes. Drain.

2. Tear the lettuce into bite-sized pieces and place in a bowl with the onion, tomatoes, olives and green beans.

3. Heat the grill. Brush the salmon steaks with a little olive oil then cook under the grill for about 2–3 minutes each side.

4. Toss the salad with the dressing. Divide into 4 bowls. Place a salmon steak on top of each. Slice the eggs into quarters and arrange next to the salmon with the lemon wedges.

Tuna and baby spinach salad

Makes 4 servings

3 peppers, 1 of each colour (red, yellow and green), thinly sliced

2 tablespoons (30 ml) chopped fresh parsley leaves

Half a red onion, thinly sliced

12 large black olives, pitted

200 g (7 oz) tuna in spring water, drained and coarsely mashed with a fork

1 pack (185 g) ready-washed baby spinach

DRESSING:

2 tablespoons (30 ml) lemon juice

3 tablespoons (45 ml) extra virgin olive oil

A little low-sodium salt, to taste

1. To make the dressing: whisk together the lemon juice, olive oil and salt in a small bowl.

2. Combine the peppers, parsley, onion, olives and tuna in a medium-size bowl. Pour the dressing over the salad and toss to coat.

3. Divide the spinach leaves among 4 plates. Top with the tuna salad. Serve immediately.

Coleslaw with hazelnuts and yoghurt dressing

Makes 4 servings

1 small white cabbage, shredded

4 medium carrots, grated

1 red onion, thinly sliced

30 g (1 oz) chopped roast hazelnuts

DRESSING:

4 tablespoons (60 ml) natural bio-yoghurt

2 teaspoons (10 ml) Dijon mustard

2 teaspoons (10 ml) low-fat mayonnaise

2 teaspoons (10 ml) lemon juice

1. In a large bowl whisk together the yoghurt, mustard, mayonnaise and lemon juice.

2. Add the cabbage, carrots, red onion and hazelnuts, tossing to combine well.

Rocket, tuna and white bean salad

Makes 4 servings

125 g (4 oz) ready-washed rocket

4 plum tomatoes, quartered

400 g (14 oz) tinned haricot or cannellini beans, drained and rinsed

200 g (7 oz) tin of tuna in spring water, drained

4 spring onions, chopped into 2.5 cm (1 in) lengths

A handful of fresh parsley, chopped

DRESSING:

2 tablespoons (30 ml) extra virgin olive oil

1 tablespoon (15 ml) lemon juice

1 clove of garlic, finely chopped

1. Place the rocket and tomatoes in a large bowl and mix together. Stir in the beans and the tuna, roughly breaking the tuna up into large flakes. Add the spring onions and parsley.

2. Shake the olive oil, lemon juice and garlic in a bottle or screw-top glass jar then drizzle over the salad. Toss well and serve.

Celery with cheese and seeds

Makes 1 serving

1 tablespoon (15 ml) low-fat soft cheese

1 teaspoon sunflower seeds, sesame seeds or pumpkin seeds

2 sticks of celery

1. Combine the soft cheese with the seeds. Spread it into the celery sticks then cut into 2.5-cm (1-inch) lengths.

2. This easy savoury snack can also be served to guests instead of crisps and salted nibbles.

Cucumber and tomato raita

Makes 300 ml (½ pint)

200 ml (7 fl oz) natural yoghurt

½ small onion, finely chopped

7.5-cm (3-inch) piece of cucumber, seeded and chopped

1 tomato, finely diced

1 teaspoon (5 ml) cumin seeds, roasted and ground*

1 tablespoon (15 ml) fresh coriander, chopped

Squeeze of lemon or lime juice

1. Place the yoghurt in a bowl. Add the onions, cucumber, tomato and cumin seeds. Stir to combine.

2. Cover and leave in the fridge until required. Serve garnished with the chopped coriander.

* To roast cumin seeds, place them on a baking sheet and roast in a preheated oven at 200° C/400° F/Gas mark 6 for 5 minutes. Crush coarsely using a pestle and mortar.

Banana and walnut loaf

100 ml (3½ fl oz) sunflower oil

2 eggs

60 ml (2 fl oz) soya, almond, oat, rice or sesame milk

225 g (8 oz) wheat-free flour

1 tablespoon (15 ml) baking powder (preferably wheat-free)

3 large ripe bananas

85 g (3 oz) walnuts, chopped

1. Preheat the oven to 180° C/350° F/Gas mark 4. Lightly oil a 500-g (1-lb) loaf tin.

2. In a large mixing bowl, beat the oil, eggs and milk until light and fluffy. Fold in the flour and baking powder.

3. Mash the bananas then add to the mixture with the walnuts. Spoon the mixture into the prepared loaf tin and bake for 1–1¼ hours until a skewer comes out clean. Turn the loaf out on to a wire rack and leave to cool.

Tofu sesame snacks

Makes 2 servings

125 g fairly firm tofu, drained and cut into bite-sized cubes

1–2 tablespoons (15–30 ml) sweet chilli sauce

2–3 tablespoons (30–45 ml) sesame seeds

Small lime or lemon wedges

1. Preheat the grill and line the grill rack with tinfoil.

2. Put the sweet chilli sauce in a bowl and the sesame seeds on a plate. Spear each tofu cube with a cocktail stick and dip them into the chilli sauce. Roll in the sesame seeds until well coated.

3. Arrange the cubes on the lined grill rack and grill the tofu for 2 minutes, or until heated through. Turn frequently during cooking to avoid burning. Garnish with lime or lemon wedges.

Cornbread

Makes 8 slices

175 g (6 oz) fine cornmeal

1 tablespoon (15 ml) wheat-free baking powder

A little low-sodium salt and freshly ground black pepper

1 egg

2 tablespoons (30 ml) olive oil

250 ml (8 fl oz) soya, almond, oat, rice or sesame milk

1. Preheat the oven to 170° C/325° F/Gas mark 3. Lightly oil a 500-g (1-lb) loaf tin.

2. Mix together the cornmeal, baking powder, low-sodium salt and pepper in a large bowl.

3. In a separate bowl combine the egg, oil and milk. Slowly add this mixture to the dry ingredients, mixing well until the mixture is smooth.

4. Pour the mixture into the prepared loaf tin and bake for 25–30 minutes until an inserted skewer comes out clean. Turn the loaf out on to a wire rack and leave to cool.

Blueberry muffins

Makes 4 servings

100 ml (3½ fl oz) rapeseed or sunflower oil

125 ml (4 fl oz) clear honey

200 ml (7 fl oz) soya, almond, oat, rice or sesame milk

1 egg

175 g (6 oz) wheat-free flour *

125 g (4 oz) fine cornmeal

1 tablespoon (15 ml) baking powder (preferably wheat-free)

150 g (5 oz) fresh or frozen blueberries

* Available from most supermarkets. Most brands contain rice flour and potato starch.

1. Preheat the oven to 200° C/ 400° F/ Gas mark 6. Line a 12-hole muffin tin with paper cases.

2. Mix together the oil, honey, milk and egg in a large jug. Sift the flour, cornmeal and baking powder into a bowl. Add the liquid mixture to the dry ingredients and stir until combined (it will be quite runny). Gently fold in the blueberries.

3. Spoon the mixture into the muffin tin and bake in the oven for 20 minutes, or until risen and golden. Leave to cool for five minutes, then transfer to a wire rack.

Creole rice with tuna

Makes 4 servings

2 tablespoons (30 ml) extra
virgin olive oil

1 onion, chopped

3 peppers (one of each colour
– red, yellow, green),

deseeded and diced

Half a chilli pepper, finely
chopped (optional)

3 large tomatoes, skinned,
chopped and deseeded

225 g (8 oz) long-grain rice

600 ml (1 pint) vegetable
stock

1 teaspoon (5 ml) fresh chives,
chopped

1 teaspoon (5 ml) fresh
parsley, chopped

A little low-sodium salt and
freshly ground black pepper,
to taste

200 g (7 oz) tinned tuna in
water, drained

1. Heat the olive oil in a heavy-
   based pan. Add the chopped
   onion and peppers and cook
   over a moderate heat for about 5
   minutes until the vegetables are
   just softened.

2. Stir in the chilli (if using),
   tomatoes and rice. Stir for 1–2
   minutes until the rice is shiny and
   coated in oil. Add the vegetable
   stock, bring to the boil then
   simmer for 25 minutes or until
   the rice is cooked.

3. Stir in the chives and parsley
   and season to taste with salt and
   pepper. Crumble the tuna into the
   rice mixture and heat through for
   a few minutes. Serve.

Chicken and red pepper risotto with spinach

Makes 4 servings

1 tablespoon (15 ml) extra virgin olive oil

1 onion, chopped

1 red pepper, deseeded and diced

300 g (10 oz) arborio (risotto) rice

1.2 litres (2 pints) hot chicken or vegetable stock

125 g (4 oz) cooked chicken, chopped

125 g (4 oz) baby spinach leaves

A little low-sodium salt and freshly ground black pepper

1. Heat the olive oil in a large heavy-based saucepan. Add the onion and red pepper and cook over a moderate heat for about 5 minutes, until the vegetables have softened.

2. Add the rice and continue cooking and stirring for 1–2 minutes, until the rice is translucent and shiny.

3. Add a ladle of the hot stock to the rice and cook, stirring constantly, over a low heat until the liquid has been absorbed. Continue adding the stock to the rice a little at a time and stirring until the liquid has been absorbed, for about 17 minutes.

4. When the rice is almost done, add the chicken and the spinach leaves and stir to mix evenly. Allow to heat through for 2–3 minutes, then adjust the seasoning to taste with low-sodium salt and pepper and serve hot.

Chestnut and vegetable burgers

Makes 4 servings

125 g (4 oz) couscous

150 ml (5 fl oz) hot vegetable stock

1 tablespoon (15 ml) extra virgin olive oil

1 onion, finely chopped

2 carrots, grated

1 courgette, finely diced

200 g (7 oz) dried chestnut pieces

1 egg, beaten

3 tablespoons (45 ml) chopped chives

A little low-sodium salt and freshly ground black pepper

Extra olive oil for brushing

1. Place the couscous in a bowl. Pour over the hot stock and leave to stand for 15 minutes until the stock has been absorbed.

2. Meanwhile, heat the oil in a frying pan and cook the onion over a moderate heat for 5 minutes. Add the carrot and courgette and continue cooking for 5 minutes. Remove from the heat.

3. Add the chestnuts, couscous, egg, chives and seasoning. Mix well.

4. Divide the mixture into 8 and firmly press into burger shapes. Chill until ready to serve.

5. Heat the grill. Place the burgers on a grill tray, brush with a little olive oil then cook for about 15 minutes, turning carefully halfway through the cooking time.

Chicken noodle salad

Makes 4 servings

1 small free-range chicken, about 1.5 kg

3 cm fresh ginger, peeled and grated

1 onion, halved

A little low-sodium salt

225 g (8 oz) rice vermicelli noodles

Half an iceberg lettuce, shredded

Half a cucumber, cut into matchstick strips

4 spring onions, chopped

4 tablespoons (60 ml) sesame seeds, toasted

DRESSING:

60 ml (2 fl oz) rice vinegar

1 tablespoon (15 ml) tahini (sesame paste) or peanut butter

2 tablespoons (30 ml) sesame oil

2 teaspoons (10 ml) soy sauce

1. Place the chicken in a large saucepan, cover with water, add the ginger, onion and low-sodium salt. Cover and bring to the boil, reduce the heat and simmer for 45 minutes.

2. Drain the chicken, remove the skin, take the meat off the bones and shred it quite finely. Discard the skin and bones.

3. Put the noodles in a bowl, cover with boiling water and let them soak for 5 minutes. Drain and rinse under cold running water.

4. Place the noodles in a large bowl. Combine with the prepared vegetables and chicken.

5. Combine the dressing ingredients in a small bowl and pour over the chicken salad. Toss to combine and sprinkle with toasted sesame seeds.

Penne with chicken and mushrooms

Makes 4 servings

300 g (10 oz) non-wheat penne pasta (or other pasta shapes)

300 g (10 oz) skinless, boneless chicken breasts

1 tablespoon (15 ml) extra virgin olive oil

2 garlic cloves, crushed

1 tablespoon (15 ml) cider vinegar

1 tablespoon (15 ml) chopped fresh tarragon

150 g (5 oz) mushrooms, sliced

150 g (5 oz) asparagus spears

1 tablespoon (15 ml) cornflour

400 ml (14 fl oz) skimmed milk (or soya, rice or oat milk)

A little low-sodium salt and freshly ground black pepper

1. Cook the penne pasta according to the packet instructions. Drain.

2. Slice the chicken into thin strips. Heat the olive oil in a heavy-based pan. Add the chicken and garlic and cook, stirring, for 5 minutes. Add the vinegar and tarragon.

3. Stir in the mushrooms and asparagus and cook for a further 2–3 minutes.

4. In a jug, blend the cornflour with a little of the milk to make a smooth paste. Stir in the remainder of the milk. Gradually add to the chicken mixture over a gentle heat, stirring continuously, until the sauce has thickened.

5. Add the sauce to the drained pasta. Mix together and serve immediately.

Florentine jackets

Makes 4 servings

2 baking (large) potatoes

225 g (8 oz) pack of ready-washed spinach leaves

125 g (4 oz) ricotta cheese

A little low-sodium salt and freshly ground black pepper

Freshly grated nutmeg

3–4 tablespoons (45–60 ml) milk

1. Preheat the oven to 200° C/ 400° F/Gas mark 6.

2. Scrub the potatoes. Prick with a fork. Place on a baking tray and bake in the oven for 1–1½ hours (depending on the size) until soft when gently pressed.

3. Place the spinach in a large saucepan with a tablespoon of water. Cover. Wilt over a low heat for a few minutes. Chop roughly and season with the low-sodium salt, black pepper and nutmeg.

4. Cut the potatoes in halves. Scoop the potato out of the skins and place in a bowl. Mash with the milk. Mix together the mashed potato, spinach and ricotta cheese.

Couscous with roasted peppers, tomatoes and mint

Makes 4 servings

2 tablespoons (30 ml) extra virgin olive oil

1 small red pepper

1 small yellow pepper

200 g (7 oz) cherry tomatoes, halved

225 g (8 oz) couscous

300 ml (½ pint) hot vegetable stock or water

400 g (14 oz) tin red kidney beans, drained and rinsed

A small handful of fresh mint, chopped

A little low-sodium salt and freshly ground black pepper

1. Preheat the oven to 200º C/ 400º F/Gas mark 6.

2. Remove the seeds from the peppers and cut them into wide strips. Place in a large roasting tin with the cherry tomatoes, drizzle over the olive oil and toss lightly so that the vegetables are well coated in the oil. Roast in the oven for about 30 minutes until the peppers are slightly charred on the outside and tender in the middle. Allow to cool then roughly chop the peppers.

3. Put the couscous in a large bowl and cover with the hot stock or water. Stir briefly, cover and allow to stand for 5 minutes until the stock has been absorbed. Fluff up with a fork.

4. Add the roast peppers, tomatoes, beans and mint. Season to taste with the low-sodium salt and black pepper. Serve.

Grilled red peppers with ricotta and basil

Makes 4 servings

4 large red peppers

175 g (6 oz) ricotta cheese

A little low-sodium salt and freshly ground black pepper

A small handful of fresh basil leaves, chopped

1–2 tablespoons (15–30 ml) extra virgin olive oil

TOMATO SAUCE:

1 tablespoon (15 ml) extra virgin olive oil

1 onion, chopped

1 garlic clove, crushed

450 g (1 lb) ripe tomatoes, skinned, deseeded and chopped, or 400 g tinned chopped tomatoes

A little low-sodium salt and freshly ground black pepper

1. Preheat the grill. Brush the peppers with a little of the olive oil, place them in a shallow tin, then place under the grill, turning frequently, until blistered and blackened all over. Put in a bowl, cover with cling film and leave to cool. Carefully remove the skin. Cut each pepper into quarters lengthways, removing the seeds. Heat the oven to 200° C/400° F/Gas mark 6.

2. Season the ricotta with low-sodium salt and pepper and mix in the basil. Take a heaped teaspoon of the mixture and place at the narrow end of each pepper. Roll up and place in an ovenproof dish.

3. Brush each pepper with olive oil and place the dish in the oven for 10 minutes.

4. Meanwhile, make the tomato sauce. Heat the olive oil in a heavy-based frying pan. Add the onion and garlic and cook over a low heat for 5 minutes until soft and transparent. Add the chopped tomatoes. Bring to the boil, reduce the heat and simmer for 10 minutes, stirring occasionally. Season with a little salt and black pepper. Serve with the grilled peppers.

Sea bass with spring vegetables

Makes 4 servings

4 x 250 g (9 oz) sea bass fillets

2 tablespoons (30 ml) extra virgin olive oil

125 g (4 oz) fine green beans, trimmed and cut into 5 cm (2 in) lengths

125 g (4 oz) sugar-snap peas, trimmed

125 g (4 oz) asparagus, trimmed and cut into 5 cm (2 in) lengths

150 g (5 oz) fresh or frozen broad beans

420 g (14 oz) tinned flageolet beans, drained and rinsed

1. Heat the oven to 180° C/ 350° F/Gas mark 4.

2. Pan-fry each sea bass fillet in the olive oil for 1 minute each side to seal, then transfer on to a baking tray and finish cooking in the oven for 8–10 minutes.

3. Steam or boil the green beans, sugar-snap peas, asparagus and broad beans for 4 minutes until they are tender-crisp. Add the flageolet beans 1 minute before the end of the cooking time so they heat through.

4. Place the sea bass in the centre of each plate then scatter the vegetables around. Serve immediately.

Breast of chicken with butternut squash mash

Makes 4 servings

4 chicken breasts on the bone

A little extra virgin olive oil

4 medium potatoes

1 butternut squash

6 tablespoons (90 ml) skimmed milk

A little low-sodium salt and freshly ground black pepper

A small handful of fresh flat-leaf parsley, chopped

1. Heat the oven to 190° C/ 375° F/Gas mark 5.

2. Scrub and prick the potatoes and cook in the oven for 45–60 minutes, depending on the size of the potatoes.

3. Meanwhile, place the chicken breasts in a roasting tin, drizzle over a little olive oil; turn the chicken so that they are well coated with oil.

4. Peel the butternut squash and cut the flesh into large chunks. Place in a separate baking tin, drizzle over a little oil and toss until well coated.

5. Cook the chicken and the squash in the oven for 20–30 minutes, depending on the size of the chicken breasts. The squash should be soft but not mushy.

6. Halve the potatoes and scoop out the flesh into a bowl. Add the cooked squash and milk, season with the salt and pepper and mash until smooth. Adjust the consistency with a little extra milk if you wish.

7. Divide the mash between four plates and place a chicken breast on top. Scatter over the chopped flat-leaf parsley and serve immediately.

Stir-fried chicken with broccoli

Makes 4 servings

2 tablespoons (30 ml) extra virgin olive oil

300 g (10 oz) chicken breasts cut into thin strips

1 tablespoon (15 ml) light (low-sodium) soy sauce

1 onion, thinly sliced

2.5 cm (1 in) piece fresh ginger, peeled and finely chopped

225 g (8 oz) broccoli florets

1 teaspoon (5 ml) cornflour blended with 1 tablespoon (15 ml) water

A handful of fresh chives, chopped

1. Heat the olive oil in a wok, add the chicken and stir-fry for 2–3 minutes until the chicken is lightly browned. Remove from the wok, place on a plate and keep warm.

2. Add the onion and ginger and stir-fry for 1 minute. Add the broccoli, continue cooking for 3 minutes, then return the chicken to the wok. Pour over the cornflour mixture, stirring continuously, until the mixture thickens.

3. Serve with cooked rice or noodles.

Fish stew with fennel and tomatoes

Makes 4 servings

2 tablespoons (30 ml) extra virgin olive oil

1 fennel bulb, finely sliced

1 garlic clove, crushed

500 ml (16 fl oz) fish or vegetable stock

800 g (18 oz) tinned chopped tomatoes

250 g (9 oz) cherry tomatoes, halved

A little low-sodium salt and freshly ground black pepper

450 g (1 lb) monkfish fillet, cut into 4 cm chunks

1 tablespoon (15 ml) chopped chives

1. Heat the olive oil in a large pan, add the fennel and cook over a moderate heat for 5 minutes. Add the garlic and cook for a further minute.

2. Stir in the stock and tinned tomatoes, bring to the boil and simmer gently for 5 minutes.

3. Add the cherry tomatoes and cook for a further 5 minutes. Season with low-sodium salt and freshly ground pepper.

4. Add the monkfish, cover and cook for approximately 5 minutes or until the fish is cooked. Serve the stew in 4 individual bowls and garnish with the chopped chives.

SHAKES, SMOOTHIES AND JUICES

Making smoothies, shakes and juices is a really easy way to meet your five a day target for fruit and vegetables. Packed with vital nutrients, they really do your body, mind and skin good. Drinks made from fresh ingredients help energise your body, detox your system, revitalise your senses and de-stress your mind.

Smoothies

- For best taste and nutritional value, choose ripe fruit.
- Remove thick peel (e.g. from bananas), stones (e.g. from peaches) and hulls (e.g. from strawberries) and cut the flesh into large chunks.
- You may substitute frozen fruit – such as raspberries – for fresh fruit.
- If your blender crushes ice, start with ice cubes blended to a 'snow' followed by the fruit. Otherwise, crush the ice before putting it into a blender.
- Add ingredients to the blender beginning with liquids and ending with solids.
- Add more or less juice or water to your smoothie, according to your own preferences, to make a thinner or thicker drink.

Melon and mint smoothie

A cupful of crushed ice

1 generous slice honeydew melon

85 ml (3 fl oz) grape or apple juice

1–2 teaspoons (5–10 ml) lemon juice

120 ml (4 fl oz) natural yoghurt

1 tablespoon (15 ml) chopped mint leaves

1. Place the ice, melon, fruit juice, lemon juice, and mint in a smoothie maker, blender or food processor and process until slushy. Serve immediately.

Shakes

- Keep the fat content low by using skimmed milk or low-fat yoghurt in the recipes.
- You may substitute soya milk or yoghurt, oat, rice or almond milk for the dairy version given in the recipes.
- For a thicker shake, add extra fruit (bananas produce the thickest creamiest consistency), crushed ice, or more yoghurt. If you use frozen fruit, the result will be a thicker drink.
- For maximum nutritional value and taste, drink your shake immediately.

Blueberry yoghurt shake

Makes 2 drinks

200 g (7 oz) blueberries

1 small banana, peeled and sliced

120 ml (4 fl oz) apple juice

150 ml (5 fl oz) natural bio-yoghurt

Crushed ice

1. Put the blueberries, banana, apple juice, bio-yoghurt and ice into a smoothie maker, blender or food processor and blend until smooth. Serve immediately.

Raspberry and cranberry shake

Makes 4 servings

A cupful of crushed ice

250 ml (8 fl oz) cranberry and raspberry juice drink

125 g (4 oz) raspberries

1 carton (150 g) natural bio-yoghurt

1. Place the ice, cranberry juice, raspberries and yoghurt in the goblet of a smoothie maker, blender or food processor and process until the ingredients are thoroughly combined. Serve immediately.

Mango and ginger shake

Makes 2 drinks

1 mango, peeled, stone removed and cut into chunks

A handful of crushed ice

2 cm (1 in) piece fresh root ginger

250 ml (8 fl oz) skimmed milk or natural bio-yoghurt

1. Put the mango flesh, ice, ginger and milk or yoghurt into a smoothie maker, blender or food processor and blend until smooth.

2. Serve immediately.

Banana, honey and almond shake

Makes 2 drinks

A cupful of crushed ice

300 ml (10 fl oz) skimmed milk

1 ripe banana

1 tablespoon (15 ml) clear honey

25 g (1 oz) ground almonds

1. Place the ice, milk, banana, almonds and honey in the goblet of a smoothie maker, blender or food processor and process until thick and frothy. Drink immediately.

Strawberry and nectarine shake

Makes 2 drinks

A cupful of crushed ice

1 carton (150 ml) strawberry bio-yoghurt

6–8 strawberries

1 nectarine, stone removed and roughly chopped

Skimmed milk

1. Put the ice, yoghurt, strawberries and nectarine in the goblet of a smoothie maker, blender or food processor and process until slushy. Adjust the consistency with skimmed milk.

2. Serve immediately.

Strawberry banana shake

Makes 4 servings

A cupful of crushed ice

125 g (4 oz) strawberries

200 ml (7 fl oz) skimmed milk

1 banana

1. Put the ice, strawberries, milk and banana in the goblet of a smoothie maker, blender or food processor and process until smooth. Adjust the consistency with milk, if necessary.

2. Serve immediately.

Orange and apricot sorbet

Makes 4 servings

300 ml (½ pint) water

125 g (4 oz) sugar

3 tablespoons (45 ml) lemon juice

Grated zest and juice of 1 large orange

400 g (14 oz) fresh apricots, halved and stoned

1 egg white

1. Put the water, sugar, lemon juice, orange zest and juice into a saucepan and bring to the boil, stirring until the sugar has dissolved. Boil rapidly for about 5 minutes. Add the apricots and simmer gently for 2 minutes. Leave to cool.

2. Pour the fruit and syrup into a food processor or blender and process to a smooth purée.

3. Pour into a container suitable for freezing, cover and freeze for about 2 hours until frozen around the sides. Alternatively, pour the mixture into an ice-cream machine and freeze until half-frozen.

4. Whisk the egg white until it forms soft peaks. If using an ice-cream maker add to the half-frozen mixture and continue freezing until completely frozen. Otherwise, tip the half-frozen mixture into a bowl and whisk briefly until smooth. Fold in the whisked egg white. Pour the mixture back into the container and freeze for about 6 hours. Remove the sorbet from the freezer about 20 minutes before serving and transfer to the fridge.

Eating on the run

When you are really busy, trying to squeeze lots of commitments into your day, it is pretty hard to stick to any healthy eating plan. However, skipped or irregular meals and hurried fatty snacks will leave you low in energy and susceptible to all the symptoms of toxicity. Here are some eating strategies to help you cope with a hectic schedule.

Plan your meal times

Always make time to eat. Plan when you will eat in advance and don't be tempted to schedule engagements at mealtimes. Fit the rest of your schedule around your mealtimes rather than the other way round.

Organise your daily food in advance

On days when you will away from home, take a supply of healthy snacks and mini-meals with you to eat (see below for ideas). That way you won't have to grab the nearest available sugary snack.

Prepare ahead

If you know that you will be pushed for time, prepare your meals in advance. For example, make a big bowl of salad or a huge pan of soup – enough for several portions. Keep the remainder in the fridge or freezer.

Shop wisely

Make a habit of shopping with a shopping list (see Chapter 4: Time for Action, pages 40–1). This saves shopping time and ensures that you will always have the right ingredients to hand in your kitchen.

Stock up

Have a stock of healthy staples in your store cupboard, so you will always be able to prepare a quick meal at short notice. Buy canned beans, lentils and tomatoes, non-wheat pasta, quinoa, millet, nuts, seeds, rye crispbreads, oatcakes and dried fruit.

Eating at work

Take healthy snacks and easy light meals with you to work. That way you won't have to rely on the choice in the canteen or local sandwich bar. Here are a few healthy ideas:

Eating on the move

It is often difficult to eat healthily when you spend a lot of your time travelling. Don't be tempted to skip meals or grab fast foods and salty snacks. Here are some ideas for healthy snacks for eating in cars, trains, buses and planes:

- Freshly squeezed juice
- Dips e.g. guacamole, hummus (see recipes, pages 70–4)
- Rye crackers, rice cakes, oatcakes
- Non-wheat bread
- Soup in a flask (see recipes, pages 78–86)
- Small packets of dried (unsulphured) fruit e.g. apricots, mangoes, sultanas
- Nuts e.g. almonds, brazils, walnuts
- Seeds e.g. sesame, sunflower
- Sesame snaps (occasional)
- A small bag of unsalted nuts, e.g. almonds, cashews
- Fresh fruit, e.g. an apple, a banana or some grapes
- Bottle of mineral water
- Mini-boxes of raisins
- Fruit bar or liquorice bar (occasional)
- Prepared vegetable sticks e.g. carrots, peppers, celery
- Rye crackers and oatcakes
- A sandwich made from rye bread

Eating out

Eating out should be enjoyable, so don't feel you have to deprive yourself and feel miserable. Don't try to stick to the diet plan completely, just choose the healthier options wherever you can. Here are some suitable choices at different types of restaurants.

Type of restaurant	Suitable Choices
Indian	Chapatti
	Chickpea dishes (e.g. channa dhal)
	Lentil dishes (e.g. dhal)
	Dry vegetable curries
	Vegetable side dishes

Chinese	Vegetable chop suey
	Stir-fried vegetables
	Rice and noodles
Italian	Pasta with tomato/ vegetable based sauces
	(e.g. Neapolitan, primavera, spinach)
	Pizza with vegetable toppings (ask to omit the cheese)
	Gnocchi with tomato-based sauce
	Pasta filled with spinach/ ricotta
	Salad with tomatoes, avocados, olives
	Vegetable risotto
Greek	Greek salad
	Tomato or cucumber salad
	Tzatziki
	Hummus
	Pitta
	Dolmades
	Stuffed tomatoes
	Fresh fruit
French	Consommé
	Ratatouille
	Salads (e.g. Niçoise)
	Vegetable dishes
	Sorbet
Mexican	Guacamole
	Bean burritos, tortillas
	Vegetable fajitas
	Tostadas with beans or vegetables
	Vegetable chilli

Try to eat healthily and lightly. A blowout meal may make you feel uncomfortable and unwell, especially if you indulge in rich food or alcohol that your body has become unaccustomed to during the detox diet. You may find that even a 'normal' meal (the kind you would eat before detoxing) is harder to digest than usual, and leaves you feeling sluggish the next day. Here are some simple tips

- Choose a vegetable or light fish main course or a main salad
- If possible, avoid meat and poultry
- Avoid rich, buttery, creamy and oily sauces
- Say no to the bread basket, especially if you are sensitive to wheat
- Add extra side salads or vegetables (oil/ vinegar dressing or olive oil are fine)
- Keep carbohydrates fairly low
- Opt for rice and potatoes instead of pasta or pizza
- Don't go for cheesy dishes, pies, quiche or anything with pastry
- Choose light fruit-based desserts
- Drink plenty of water
- Set yourself a sensible alcohol limit (say, 1–2 glasses of wine)
- Have herbal tea (e.g. peppermint or camomile) instead of coffee

Family meals

There is no need to prepare separate meals for yourself and the rest of your family. In fact, the whole family can benefit from the detox diet. Many of the meals and recipes can easily be adapted to suit the needs and tastes of other family members. You can increase their portion sizes and add a few extras, such as poultry, fish or low-fat dairy products, to meet their requirements. You may find that your other half becomes a willing convert!

However, this detox diet is unsuitable for children under 18 because they are still growing and developing.

Feeding your children

Young children have high calorie and nutritional needs relative to their smaller body size. They cannot cope with large volumes of fibre-rich foods so don't expect them to eat the same amount of vegetables, fruits and pulses as you. They will require more protein, vitamins, calcium and iron.

However, children can still benefit from a diet that emphasises fruit, vegetables, nuts, pulses and seeds. So introduce some of the recipes in Chapter 6 into your family meal repertoire, adjusting the portion sizes and adding a little extra protein (e.g. poultry, fish, dairy products) and other cereals (e.g. ordinary bread and cereals).

CHAPTER 8

NUTRITION AND SUPPLEMENT GUIDE

The 28 day detox diet should be the start of a lifelong pattern of healthy eating. This chapter tells you how to put together a balanced diet that ensures you get all the nutrients your body needs. It also gives you more detail about the supplements you should be taking and provides a guide to helpful foods and supplements for various common ailments. During the 28 day detox diet – and beyond – you should select a wide variety of foods from each food group to get the right amount of energy, protein, carbohydrate, fibre, fats and oils, vitamins, minerals, phytochemicals and antioxidants. Here's a quick guide:

Protein

Protein is needed for cell growth and repair. It is also used to make hormones, enzymes and antibodies. There are many different types of proteins, all of which are made up of amino acids, which can be combined together in different ways. Eight of these amino acids cannot be made in the body and must come from your food. Foods that supply good amounts of all eight essential amino acids (EAAs) include meat, fish, dairy products, soya and eggs. Since these are not permitted during the 28 day detox diet, you should make sure that you include a variety of plant-based proteins in your daily diet: pulses, whole grains, nuts and seeds. These foods supply smaller amounts of EAAs and may be lacking in one or two, so you need to combine two or more of these foods to get the right balance. Suitable combinations include the following:

- Red lentils and brown rice
- Hummus (chickpea dip) and oatcakes
- Quinoa with almonds and sesame seeds

Carbohydrate

Carbohydrate is your body's main fuel and should supply around half of your daily calories. Some carbohydrate foods are 'slow-releasing' (i.e. they produce a gradual rise in blood sugar), which means that they produce sustained energy. These foods mainly include whole grains, pulses, vegetables and fresh fruit.

Other carbohydrates, including sugary foods and drinks and most refined foods, are 'fast-releasing', producing a rapid rise in blood sugar. These are best kept to a minimum. If you rely on lots of fast-releasing carbohydrates you may get large swings in blood-sugar levels, which can lead to problems with blood-sugar control, such as hypoglycaemia.

On the detox diet, you should eat mostly slow-releasing carbohydrates. Fast-releasing carbohydrate foods, such as potatoes or rice cakes, should be combined with a protein food or an oily food, for example a baked potato with a little olive oil, or a rice cake spread with hummus. Always choose unrefined carbohydrates – wholegrain cereals, brown rice, and jacket potatoes – as these will give you plenty of fibre, vitamins and minerals. Fibre helps to keep your gut healthy, allowing food to pass through the body and preventing constipation. It also helps slow the absorption of digested carbohydrate into the blood and maintains good energy levels.

Fats and oils

A certain amount of fat or oil is needed in the diet. This helps you absorb the fat-soluble vitamins A, D and E and is the only source of the essential fatty acids (EFAs). However, fats are the most concentrated sources of calories, and should make up no more than 30 per cent of your daily calorie intake. The most beneficial types of fat are the EFAs. These are vital for health and cannot be made in your body so they must be supplied in your diet.

There are two families of EFAs, the omega-3 oils and the omega-6 oils. You need both to be healthy but most people get too little omega-3 in relation to omega-6. Oily fish, flaxseeds (linseeds), pumpkinseeds and walnuts are the best sources of omega-3s. Most other seed (vegetable) oils, nuts, seeds and whole grains are rich in omega-6s. But it's the omega-3s that give so many health benefits. For example they do
the following:

- Reduce risk of heart attacks and strokes.
- Help lower blood fats.
- Reduce joint stiffness and pain.
- Alleviate rheumatoid arthritis.
- Improve oxygen delivery to your cells.
- Indirectly help your weight-loss efforts.

In fact, so strong is the evidence for omega-3s that the Department of Health recommends eating at least one portion of oily fish per week. While on the detox diet, you can get the same benefits by eating 2 to 4 tablespoons of flaxseeds (milled) or up to 4 tablespoons of an essential oil blend.

Vitamins and minerals

Vitamins and minerals are substances that are needed in tiny amounts to enable your body to work properly and ward off diseases. There are many different vitamins which are needed to support almost every system in the body, including your immune system, nervous system and hormonal system. The minerals have mainly structural roles (such as calcium in the bones) or regulatory roles (e.g. fluid balance, muscle contraction). The chart on pages 210–12 tells you more about the functions and food sources of the key vitamins and minerals.

While your diet should supply you with most of your vitamin and mineral requirements, you may need extra help in the form of multivitamin and mineral supplements. These act as an insurance policy against possible low intakes, particularly if you are under stress, smoke, drink alcohol, exercise regularly, or cannot always eat a balanced diet. A supplement may also give you added protection from disease in later life.

The most beneficial nutrients in this respect are the antioxidant nutrients, such as vitamins C and E and selenium. Some experts also claim that higher intakes of vitamins and minerals will promote and maintain optimal health. This, they say, will allow you to perform better both physically and mentally, to resist infections more effectively and even to extend your lifespan.

When selecting a supplement, choose a brand that provides between 100 and 1000 per cent of the recommended daily amount (RDA) of all the vitamins and around 100 per cent of the RDA of the minerals. Try to choose brands that have been produced by established manufacturers with a good reputation for quality control and clinical research.

Phytochemicals

Phytochemicals are plant compounds that are beneficial for your health. You get them from fruit, vegetables, grains, pulses, soya products and herbs. Many phytochemicals work as antioxidants (see below), while others influence enzymes (such as those that block cancer agents). They have the following benefits:

- Fight cancer.
- Reduce inflammation.
- Combat free radicals.
- Lower cholesterol.
- Reduce heart disease risk.
- Boost immunity.
- Balance gut bacteria.
- Fight harmful bacteria and viruses.

For the best protection, eat a mainly plant-food diet and include a wide variety of different coloured foods. In general, the more intensely coloured the fruit or vegetable, the greater the concentration of phytochemicals, vitamins and minerals.

You can maximise your phytochemical mix by choosing foods from each colour category every day:

- Green – watercress, broccoli, cabbage, rocket, Brussels sprouts, salad leaves, curly kale
- Red/ purple – plums, aubergine, cherries, beetroot, red grapes, strawberries, blackberries, blueberries, tomatoes
- Yellow/ orange – peaches, apricots, nectarines, oranges, yellow peppers, squash
- White/ yellow – onions, garlic, apples, pears, celery

Antioxidants

Antioxidants are substances that protect your body from the effects of free radical damage. They include enzymes, vitamins (such as beta-carotene, vitamin C, vitamin E), minerals (such as selenium) and phytochemicals (such as flavanoids). Without antioxidants your body would eventually 'rust'! Free radicals are produced all the time as a normal part of cell processes.

In small numbers they are not a problem. But extra free radicals can be generated by pollution, UV sunlight, cigarette smoke and stress. Left unchecked, they can fur up your arteries, and increase your risk of thrombosis, heart disease and cancer.

The good news is that an antioxidant-rich diet may help protect against these conditions and slow the ageing process. Antioxidant nutrients are found in fruit and vegetables, seed oils, nuts, whole grains and pulses: just about all the foods permitted in the 28 day detox diet!

The fruits and vegetables with the highest antioxidant power include: prunes; raisins; blueberries; blackberries; garlic; curly kale; strawberries; raspberries; spinach; Brussels sprouts; plums; alfalfa sprouts; red peppers; broccoli.

Nutritional supplements

1. Antioxidants

WHAT THEY DO
Beta-carotene is a powerful free radical scavenger that destroys carcinogens (cancer-causing substances), guards against heart disease and strokes and lowers cholesterol levels. Vitamin C detoxifies many harmful substances and plays a key role in immunity. It increases a natural antiviral substance produced by the body and stimulates the activity of key immune cells. Vitamin E is a powerful antioxidant that prevents the cells from becoming rancid as a result of free radicals. It also improves oxygen utilisation, enhances your immune response and plays a role in the prevention of cataracts caused by free radical damage.

HOW TO USE THEM
One supplement taken daily containing around 15 to 25 mg of beta-carotene, up to 1000 mg of vitamin C, 250 to 500 mg of vitamin E plus a range of other antioxidant nutrients.

2. Kelp

WHAT IT DOES
- Extremely rich source of iodine, iron, calcium and zinc.
- Helps the function of the thyroid gland, which in turn controls your metabolic rate.

- May help weight loss.
- Beneficial to brain tissue, the membranes surrounding the brain, the sensory nerves and the spinal chord as well as the nails and blood vessels.
- Useful for hair loss, obesity and ulcers.

HOW TO USE IT
One tablet of kelp a day, containing no more than 250 micrograms of iodine.

3. Milk Thistle

WHAT IT DOES

- Protects liver cells from the effects of alcohol and other toxins.
- Stimulates the production of new liver cells.
- Improves liver function.
- Protects the kidneys.
- Good for inflammatory bowel disorders and a weakened immune system.
- Beneficial for psoriasis and skin problems.

HOW TO USE IT
Take up to 420 mg of standardised silymarin (milk thistle) capsules per day.

4. Essential oil blend

WHAT IT DOES

- Increases your energy levels.
- Speeds fat loss.
- Benefits your heart and cardiovascular health.
- Boosts immune function.

HOW TO USE IT
Take 1 to 4 tablespoons a day.

5. Spirulina

WHAT IT DOES

- Provides key nutrients such as protein, vitamins, potassium, phosphorus, iron, manganese and zinc, which help to cleanse and regenerate tissues.
- Helps to regenerate and purify the blood.

HOW TO USE IT
No more than 3 g a day unless otherwise directed.

6. Chlorella

Chlorella is used by leading dentists to support the detoxification of heavy metal toxicity.

WHAT IT DOES

- The chlorophyll in chlorella can speed up the cleansing process of the bloodstream.
- Bio available sources of protein, B vitamins including B12, vitamins C and E, amino acids and wide spectrum minerals.
- High in RNA and DNA and protects against the effects of ultra-violet radiation.
- Beneficial for non-meat eaters.

HOW TO USE IT
No more than 3 g a day unless otherwise directed.

The Essential Vitamins and Minerals Guide

Vitamin	Needed for:	Best food sources
A	Vision in dim light; healthy skin and linings of the digestive tract, nose and throat	Full fat dairy products e.g. meat, offal, oily fish, margarine, parsley, peas, whole grains, legumes
Beta-carotene	Antioxidant which protects against certain cancers and converts into vitamin A	Fruit and vegetables e.g. apricots, peppers, tomatoes, mangoes, broccoli, squash, carrots, watercress
Vitamin B1 (Thiamin)	Release of energy from carbohydrates, healthy nerves and the digestive system	Wholemeal bread and cereals, pulses, meat, sunflower seeds
Vitamin B2 (Riboflavin)	Release of energy from carbohydrates, healthy skin, eyes and nerves	Milk and dairy products (organic; goat's or sheep's), meat, eggs, soya products, leafy green vegetables, avocado, whole grains
Vitamin B3 (Niacin)	Release of energy from carbohydrates, healthy skin, nerves and digestion	Meat and offal, fish, nuts, milk and dairy products, eggs, whole-grain cereals, dates, alfalfa
Vitamin B6 (Pyridoxine)	Metabolism of protein, carbohydrate and fat, manufacture of red blood cells, healthy immune system	Pulses, nuts, eggs, cereals, fish, bananas, sunflower seeds

Vitamin	Needed for:	Best food sources
Folic Acid	Formation of DNA and red blood cells, reduces risk of spina bifida in developing babies	Green leafy vegetables, yeast extract, pulses, nuts, citrus fruit
Vitamin B12	Formation of red blood cells, energy metabolism	Milk and dairy products, meat, fish, fortified breakfast cereals, soya products, yeast extract, alfalfa, sea vegetables
Vitamin C	Healthy connective tissue, bones, blood vessels, gums and teeth. Promotes immune function and helps iron absorption	Fruit and vegetables e.g. raspberries, blackcurrants, kiwi, oranges, peppers, broccoli, cabbage, tomatoes
Vitamin D	Builds strong bones: needed to absorb sunlight, calcium and phosphorus	Oily fish, fortified margarine, cold pressed vegetable oil, breakfast cereals, eggs, parsley, alfalfa
Vitamin E	Antioxidant which helps protect against heart disease, promotes normal cell growth and development	Cold pressed vegetable/ seed oils, oily fish, nuts, seeds, egg yolk, avocado, brown rice
Calcium	Building bone and teeth, blood clotting, nerve and muscle function	Milk and dairy products, sardines, dark green leafy vegetables, pulses, brazil nuts, almonds, figs, and sesame seeds

Vitamin	Needed for:	Best food sources
Iron	Formation of red blood cells and oxygen transport. Prevents anaemia	Meat and offal, whole-grain cereals, fortified breakfast cereals, pulses, green leafy vegetables, nuts, sesame and pumpkinseeds
Zinc	Healthy immune system, wound healing, skin, cell growth	Eggs, whole-grain cereals, meat, nuts and seeds
Magnesium	Healthy bones, muscle and nerve function and cell formation	Cereals, fruit, vegetables, milk, nuts and seeds
Potassium	Fluid balance, muscle and nerve function	Fruit, vegetables, cereals, nuts and seeds
Sodium	Fluid balance, muscle and nerve function	Salt, processed meat, ready meals, sauces, soup, cheese, bread
Selenium	Antioxidant which helps protect against heart disease and cancer	Cereals, vegetables, dairy products, meat, eggs, nuts and seeds

Ready reckoner

A number of common ailments can be prevented or alleviated through diet and use of supplements. However, if you have a medical condition you should seek professional medical advice. Always follow the recommendations on the packet of whatever supplement you choose.

Condition	Helpful foods	Helpful supplements
POOR IMMUNITY You are susceptible to colds and viruses	Foods rich in phyto-chemicals and anti-oxidants: citrus fruit,	Vitamin C Antioxidant supplement Zinc lozenges

Condition	Helpful foods	Helpful supplements
	all berries, dark green leafy vegetables, garlic, carrots, seeds and nuts	Garlic capsules Echinacea Golden seal root
CONSTIPATION You have infrequent bowel movements	Fibre-rich foods: whole grains, all fruit and vegetables, nuts, flax-seeds, sunflower seeds, chickpeas. Water: 6 to 8 glasses daily	Psyllium husks Aloe vera Dandelion root
IRRITABLE BOWEL SYNDROME You may have alternating, constipation/ diarrhoea abdominal pain, cramping and bloating.	Foods rich in probiotic (friendly) bacteria: live bio yoghurt, fermented milk or yoghurt drinks (containing lactobacilli). Foods rich in fructo-oligosaccharides: Jerusalem artichokes, bananas, garlic, onions, asparagus, barley and wheat	Probiotic supplements Fish oil supplements Evening primrose oil Peppermint supplements Chlorella
INSOMNIA You find it difficult to get a good night's sleep	Tryptophan-containing foods, such as turkey, chicken, cauliflower, broccoli, dairy products, lean meat, fish, eggs, and soya products. Base evening meal on carbohydrate foods, such as pasta, potatoes, rice and fruit with a small amount of protein, such as fish, poultry, and pulses. Avoid caffeine-containing drinks – choose peppermint, camomile,	Valerian Passiflora Melissa officinalis (extract of hops) Lemon balm High-strength multivitamins

Condition	Helpful foods	Helpful supplements
	lemon balm or valerian teas. Foods rich in B vitamins and magnesium: whole grains, pulses, nuts	
FATIGUE You feel tired all the time and have difficulty concentrating	Iron-rich foods: pulses, nuts, seeds, green leafy vegetables, and wheat germ. Accompany with vitamin C-rich food or drink e.g. freshly squeezed citrus juice, berries, oranges, green leafy vegetables. Foods rich in B vitamins: whole grains, pulses, seeds, nuts. Magnesium-rich foods: nuts, dark green leafy vegetables, fish, seeds, whole grain bread and cereals	Multivitamin and mineral supplements (containing 15 mg iron, B vitamins, magnesium, zinc) Spirulina
SKIN PROBLEMS You have a tendency to dry skin, itchiness, flakiness, or mild acne	Foods rich in beta-carotene: orange, red and green fruit and vegetables. Nuts, seeds, avocados and whole grains for vitamin E and zinc. Foods rich in essential fatty acids: flaxseeds, pumpkinseeds, blended essential oil, flaxseed/pumpkinseed and walnut/sesame oil. 6 to 8 glasses of water	Evening primrose oil capsules

INDEX